THE DIET *Alternative*

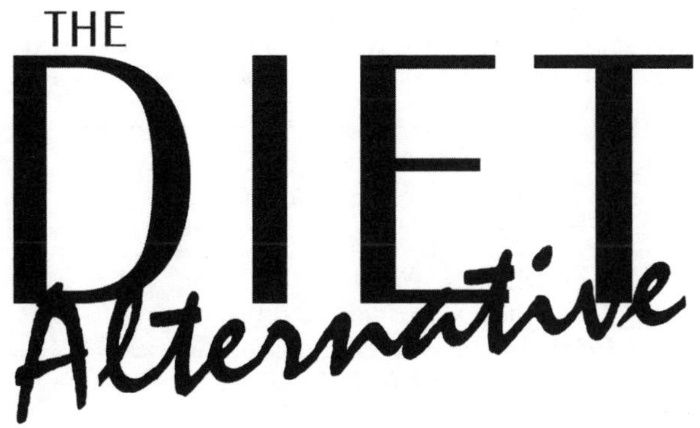

Diane Hampton

WHITAKER
HOUSE

This book is not intended to provide medical advice or to take the place of medical advice and treatment from your personal physician. Readers are advised to consult their own doctors or other qualified health professionals regarding the treatment of their medical problems and before undertaking any change in their physical regimen, whether fasting, diet, or exercise. Neither the publisher nor the author takes any responsibility for any possible consequences from any treatment to or action taken by any person reading or following the information in this book.

THE DIET ALTERNATIVE
Revised Version with Study Guide

ISBN-13: 978-0-88368-721-5
ISBN-10: 0-88368-721-6
Printed in the United States of America

Whitaker House
1030 Hunt Valley Circle
New Kensington, PA 15068
www.whitakerhouse.com

Library of Congress Cataloging-in-Publication Data

Hampton, Diane.
The diet alternative / Diane Hampton.
p. cm.
ISBN 0-88368-721-6 (alk. paper)
1. Dieters—Religious life. 2. Compulsive eaters—Religious life. 3. Obesity—Religious aspects—Christianity. 4. Gluttony. I. Title.
BV4596.D53 H36 2002
261.8'3225—dc21 2001008398

---

2 3 4 5 6 7 8 9 10 11 12 ꟽ 14 13 12 11 10 09 08 07

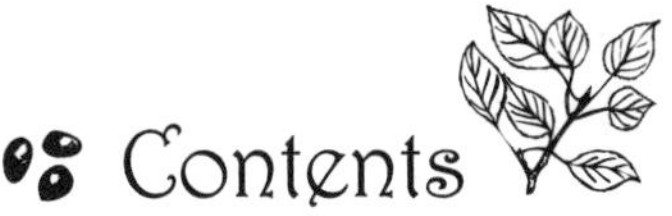

Contents

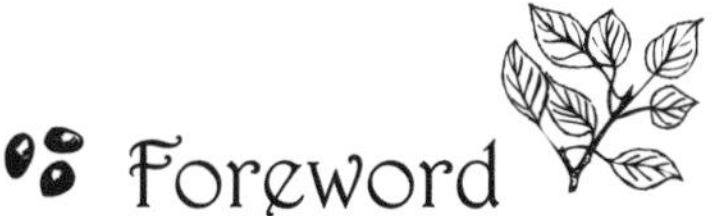

Foreword

Can people be freed from bondages that they have struggled with for most of their lives?

Is their help, which they may never have dreamed of, possible?

Is it too late to begin again?

This is a book about experiencing the freedom that God has made available through His Son, Jesus Christ.

It is power-packed with truth and fresh insight that can change your life.

If you are experiencing anything less than freedom in any area of your life, you *can* have freedom.

"Therefore if the Son makes you free, you shall be free indeed" (John 8:36).

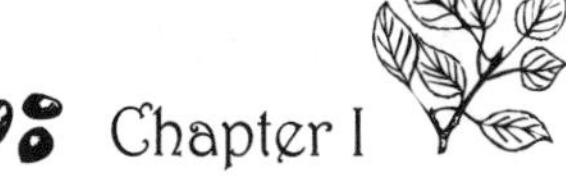

Chapter I
Deliverance from Gluttony

I can still remember going to my personal physician some twenty-plus years ago. I was deeply involved in binge eating, and I had such a feeling of desperation watching my weight go up and up as it had so many times before. I knew that it was out of control, but I didn't know how to get that control back.

I remember explaining to my doctor what I was going through and how frightened I was. After listening to me for a few minutes, he left the room and came back with a 1000-calorie-a-day diet. How could he have had so little understanding! *If I could have stayed on a diet, I wouldn't have had a weight problem!* I knew how many calories there were in everything I ate. But knowing that still didn't stop me from overeating.

Desperate!

Once, I gained thirty pounds in three months. Food was on my mind constantly. When I woke up in the morning, my first thoughts were about what I would eat that day. I wondered if I would be able to control my eating at all, or if I would succumb to my desire to gorge. Even when I was on one of my frequent diets (periodically I was able to reach my normal weight and maintain it for a few months), I was obsessed with thoughts of food. I was also often depressed.

I read every diet and weight-control book I could find. I tried self-hypnosis. I went to a physician for hypnosis. I went to a psychologist. I even went to a weight doctor. *But there was something inside me that continued to drive me to overeat.*

Experiencing Sin's Control

If you substitute the words *eating* and *overeating* for sin and wrongdoing in Paul's letter to the Romans, you have a good explanation of what it's like to be a compulsive eater. Even more important, you see what it takes to overcome it.

> *I don't understand myself at all, for I really want to do* [eat] *what is right, but I can't. I do* [eat] *what I don't want to—what I hate* [a person will eat almost anything on a binge]. *I know perfectly well that what I am doing* [overeating] *is wrong, and my bad conscience proves that I agree with these laws I am breaking* [condemnation is a constant companion of a compulsive eater]. *But I can't help myself, because I'm no longer doing it. It is sin inside me that is stronger than I am that makes me do these evil things* [this overeating].
>
> *I know I am rotten through and through so far as my old sinful nature is concerned. No matter which*

> *way I turn* [psychology, hypnosis, crash diets] *I can't make myself do right* [eat right]. *I want to but I can't. When I want to do good* [try to diet], *I don't* [I eat anyway]; *and when I try not to do wrong* [overeat], *I do it anyway. Now if I am doing what I don't want to, it is plain where the trouble is: sin still has me in its evil grasp.*
>
> (Romans 7:15–20 TLB)

"Oh, what a terrible predicament I'm in! Who will free me from my slavery to this deadly overeating?" (See verse 24.)

How You Can Be Free

"Thank God! Jesus Christ our Lord did! He has set me free!" (See Romans 7:25.)

> *So there is now no condemnation awaiting those who belong to Christ Jesus. For the power of the life-giving Spirit—and this power is mine through Christ Jesus—has freed me from the vicious circle of sin and death* [overeating and guilt]. *We aren't saved from sin's grasp by knowing the commandments of God* [how to diet], *because we can't and don't keep them, but God put into effect a different plan to save us. He sent his own Son in a human body like ours—except that ours are sinful—and destroyed sin's* [overeating's] *control over us by giving himself as a sacrifice for our sins* [overeating]. *So now we can obey God's laws* [overcome overeating] *if we follow after the Holy Spirit and no longer obey the old evil nature within us.*
>
> (Romans 8:1–4 TLB)

I remember, as a binge eater, looking at people who never had a weight problem. I could not even imagine what it felt like not to be concerned with and controlled by food. I remember reading an article about Johnny Carson where he made a statement about not really caring what he ate.

He said he ate because it was something he had to do. It was impossible for me to relate to that statement. I remember thinking what a strange remark that was and wondering if that was how it felt to be in control of your eating.

Free at Last

Now, after being completely healed for over twenty years, I know what control feels like. Sometimes it is hard for me to remember what it was like as a glutton or food addict because God put my shame *"as far as the east is from the west."* That's how *"far has He removed our transgressions from us"* (Psalm 103:12).

Today I can think of hundreds of things I would rather do than eat. I often get busy during the day and realize about 4:00 PM that I haven't eaten all day. Then I realize, I'm really hungry! I enjoy food much more now because there is no condemnation when I eat. It is amazing how much better food tastes when you are genuinely hungry.

One thing I really enjoy is throwing out leftover cake or pie. I guess you have to have been a binge eater to really appreciate this experience. In the past, these things would always have been eaten, often in one day! Right now we are eating a box of chocolates that was given to us a month ago.

Now that is freedom!

Jesus said, *"Therefore if the Son makes you free, you shall be free indeed"* (John 8:36). I now have freedom to have one chocolate instead of half a box or two or three chocolate chip cookies instead of a dozen. I am free indeed!

Another new and wonderful experience is not changing dress sizes. At every change of season, I had clothes I could not wear. They were either too big or too small because my size was constantly changing. I haven't changed dress sizes in twenty years.

In these past twenty years, my family has undergone many changes. I have watched our young daughters grow into beautiful brides with husbands of their own.

My family isn't the only thing that has changed. Life itself is dramatic. It cannot be controlled, and it sometimes takes unexpected turns. My husband has a very successful engineering company. He has spent his lifetime building it up to be an excellent company that provides employment for many families.

Suddenly—literally overnight—it was all under eleven feet of filthy, stinking floodwater in the Great Floods of 1993. It appeared that we had lost everything. Without any flood insurance, we had no hope of recovering.

But when we looked to Jesus, He gave us hope. He said, *"With men it is impossible* [that fit our situation], *but not with God; for with God all things are possible"* (Mark 10:27). We had something much better than insurance coverage: we had a wonderful promise from God's Word. God turned our losses into gain and, within a couple of years, my husband's company was named one of the top ten engineering companies in the United States in the area of their expertise.

Sometimes it seems as if the more difficult the situation, the more hopeless it looks and feels, the more good God brings. I don't understand it, I can't comprehend it, and I never see a possible way that good could be brought from some of the messes of life, but *God does it.* I have learned to *"know"* this as Paul did: *"And we know* [we have learned from lots and lots of experiences] *that all things* [ALL things] ***work together for good to those who love God,*** *to those who are the called according to His purpose"* (Romans 8:28, emphasis added).

God *always* has an answer because He is God. Just because we can't see an answer doesn't mean that there is no answer. Our minds go round and round in perplexing circles of anxiety, seeking an answer that we can't find.

We don't see what God sees or know what God knows. He isn't wringing His holy hands and pacing the golden streets of heaven. He doesn't ask us to solve the problem, but He does ask things of us. He asks us to *"believe"* and not to allow our hearts to *"be troubled* [be filled with anxiety and fear]" (John 14:1). When we do these things, we do what is right, as well. As we believe, we keep our actions and hearts in the right place for Him to work His miracles. *"Let not your heart be troubled; you believe in God, believe also in Me"* (John 14:1). *"This is the work of God, that you believe in Him whom He sent"* (John 6:29).

God doesn't just put a Band-Aid on a problem. He solves it, restores it, or even recreates it. Not once have any fear-producing circumstances turned me back to food. Food has lost its power over me, and I am ever growing closer to the place where I *"count it all joy"* when trials come (James 1:2). I'm not there yet, but I am ever closer. There is only *one* reason for this change, and it is God's deep faithfulness.

These challenges only make us stronger in Christ Jesus our Lord. It never seems like it at the time, but I have learned that God is always faithful when we keep our eyes on Him.

The Source of Healing Never Changes

The wonderful healing from compulsive eating has lasted. That awful, nagging urge to overeat is gone. Bodies change through the decades. Ages thirty-five, forty-five, and fifty-five are times when bodies experience physical changes that will gradually cause a slow, but steady, weight gain if no adjustment is made. It happens even if a person does not increase her food intake.

Several times I found that I needed to make adjustments because my body was changing. It was so simple when I wasn't driven to eat. I have always gone back to the One who has all the answers. I have a sure knowledge that my healing came from my relationship with God, not some legalistic regime that was set in stone.

Each communion with the Holy Spirit has gently impressed small changes that I could incorporate into my life. Each insight has allowed me to continue to maintain my weight and dress size while improving my health and energy at the same time.

Most people guess my age to be ten or fifteen years younger than I actually am. I have found that in Christ—in that relationship with our Savior—*"are hidden all the treasures of wisdom and knowledge"* (Colossians 2:3).

I'll never stop thanking God for sending Jesus to save me from the gluttony and depression that was robbing me of my freedom and joy. No one can imagine all the wonderful experiences God has planned for our lives in Christ. The joy of being free has allowed me to serve others and focus on God's plans and purposes for my life in a much more meaningful way.

God brings light into our lives. I remember, when I had been binge eating and someone came to the door, the feeling of not wanting to be with other people. I felt as if they somehow knew I had been overeating. There was always that hidden part of me, that darkness, that only I knew about. Now there is no more darkness inside me, no hidden shame.

Are You Born Again?

Jesus said, *"Unless one is born of water and the Spirit, he cannot enter the kingdom of God"* (John 3:5). It is possible that you have not experienced what God has made available to you.

What does it mean to be "born again"? I was born again late one night when I was all alone. I had been reading the Bible for the first time in my life. Although I attended church every week and recited a creed that expressed the truth, I had no real relationship with God. I had never been born again. I didn't even know what that expression meant! Like Nicodemus, I would hear those words and think, "What does that mean? How can a person be born again?" (See John 3:4.)

It means that your spirit comes alive to God, and you can come to know your Creator, God the Father. It means that you have been delivered from one kind of life (in the flesh) into another kind of life (in the Spirit). One is marked by fear and bondage, and the other is marked by love and freedom. One is subject to death, and the other is subject to life. One is subject to lies, deceptions, and a hundred false starts. The other is subject to truth, answers, and fruitful new beginnings that bring wonderful changes.

When I was born again, I wasn't instantly healed of my binge eating and food addiction. However, I was now in a position to receive God's help and wisdom. As a new believer, I just wanted to lose weight and be freed from that darkness of depression.

Yet God wanted to give me a new life! He had so much more for me than I had ever dared hope.

Freedom from Bondage

I recently had a young man working at my home. He was complaining that he hadn't gotten to sleep until 4:30 AM. He said, "I just can't sleep." It was a bondage in his life. He could not free himself. He went outside to begin working, but his words kept coming back to me. I remembered what it was like to have trouble sleeping. There was that awful, empty place inside me. Life had no meaning or purpose. I often lay awake thinking about death.

I felt the Holy Spirit begin to gently urge me to speak to this young man about Jesus. The question came up in my spirit, "Why do you think he can't sleep?" I knew why he couldn't sleep. He was afraid of death. The Bible puts it this way in the book of Hebrews. Jesus died to *"release those who through fear of death were all their lifetime subject to bondage"* (Hebrews 2:15).

I finally walked outside to where he was working. Again the Holy Spirit was reaching out to him through me. "Ask him if he ever thinks about God." I felt awkward and unsure of myself, but the inward witness was growing stronger. Finally, I said, "Do you ever think about God?"

He stopped his work and didn't speak for a long moment. Then he said, very slowly and very quietly, "As a matter of fact, I do think about God."

Within a very short period of time, this young man was asking Jesus Christ to be his Savior and to forgive him for all his sins. He was "born again." His spirit was now alive to God, and he was able to begin a loving relationship with his Father in heaven. I have kept in close touch with this young man. Last week he was pretty frustrated because an old friend had called him at 1:30 AM. He was frustrated because the phone call had awakened him from a sound sleep. That awful bondage of not being able to sleep was gone because he had a restored relationship with his Creator. The Holy Spirit wants to open prison doors, to release those who are bound, and to heal broken hearts. (See Isaiah 61:1.)

Jesus said, *"Unless one is born again, he cannot see the kingdom of God"* (John 3:3). He cannot experience or benefit from the kingdom of God. In a very real way, that person is separated from life. He has a strong witness inside that something is missing—he has a sense of purposelessness, hopelessness, and lack of meaning.

God Has Made a Way

If you want to be "born again," you don't need anyone else there with you because God is waiting for you with open arms! You can pray in your own words, from a sincere heart that is desperate to be free and humble enough to acknowledge that you are a sinner. You want to be able to live your life differently, but you need help. You feel something inside you that gives witness that Jesus Christ is the

Son of God. With that belief in your heart, you speak from your mouth. "Father, I feel lost and afraid. I know I have done wrong things, and I would give anything to start all over again. I believe that You have made this possible through Your Son, Jesus Christ. I am asking You now, Father, to forgive my sins, in Jesus' name, and bring me into everlasting life. I receive it now, in Jesus' name. Amen."

When you do this sincerely, you will be born again. The Bible will become different to you. You will be able to understand many of the things that Jesus talked about. God has a wonderful plan for your life that you can now begin to walk out with His help and love. Best of all, you will be able to receive the healing power that this book talks about.

God's wonderful plan for your life will begin to unfold. When you realize who Jesus is and what He did for you, your whole life can be changed. *"Old things have passed away; behold, all things have become new"* (2 Corinthians 5:17). When I was born again, Scriptures that I had heard almost all my life became real to me. Jesus became the Lord of my life. His death and resurrection, which saved me from my sins, became exciting to me because it was personal! I found a Source for my life, a Teacher, a Word that was Truth itself and would never change or let me down. I found a place to take this awful torment inside me.

A New Life

I am thankful that the weight did not just drop off because someone laid hands on me and prayed, although I do thank God for His supernatural intervention in our lives. I didn't just lose weight; I found a new way of life! I learned that Jesus is truly *"able to keep* [me] *from stumbling, and to present* [me] *faultless before the presence of His glory with exceeding joy"* (Jude 24). I learned that God's Word is true, and I learned how to apply it to my life and receive healing. Because of this, I have found "exceeding joy" that does not diminish.

The Lord is more real to me today than He was that night over twenty years ago. He continues to be my Savior.

As long as we live on this earth, *Satan will never stop trying to gain a foothold in our lives, but Jesus will never stop being our Savior from all sin.* As long as we choose Jesus, sin will have no power over us.

Gluttony is a spiritual problem. Until that "spirit of overeating" is gone, you will never live in lasting victory over your weight. Conversely, once that "spirit of overeating" is gone, eating will never again be a problem in your life.

Chapter 2

Spiritual Battles Have Spiritual Answers

Binge eating, compulsive eating, bulimia, and other eating disorders are spiritual in their origin and have a spiritual solution. Even outside the Christian community, this fact is acknowledged. I was once talking to a woman who worked in the psychiatric unit of a well-known hospital. It had a residential treatment program for drug and alcohol abuse and eating disorders. She said, "There are no programs for these addictions anywhere that don't include God." In other words, there is something at work in these addictions that is spiritual. Teen Challenge has the highest success rate in the world in treating drug and alcohol addictions, and its program is spiritual (Christian).

The desire to gorge, purge, or starve seems almost like a living thing inside a person. Eventually, it can grow until it controls our lives. It can become what the Bible calls *"strongholds"* (2 Corinthians 10:4). What is a stronghold? It's something that has a *strong hold* on some area of a person's life. It is an unbreakable, destructive habit that is the opposite of freedom. Actually, in varying degrees, it controls a great deal of a person's life. It controls or strongly influences what they do, what they think, how they spend their money, how they perceive themselves, and how they treat others.

Food addictions are only one of a plethora of bondages. Some are as minor as a compulsion toward diet soda. Some are as serious as pornography, destructive drugs, cancer-producing smoking, gambling, and other things that begin to have power over our own wills.

The freedom that we can have through God brings opposite results. God develops constructive choices that bring us into a place of peace and rest, where we become forces for good in this world. Rather than containing secret shame, our lives become full of light that can draw others to God.

Fighting Flesh with Flesh Equals Failure

Jesus said, *"It is the Spirit who gives life; the flesh profits* ***nothing****. The words that I speak to you are spirit, and they are life"* (John 6:63, emphasis added). Jesus is telling us that flesh cannot overcome flesh. That is why nearly every women's magazine regularly runs front-cover headlines about the newest absolutely, positively, "sure-fire" way to lose weight and keep it off. New diets constantly come on the market because the old ones don't seem to work or bring lasting results. Most overweight people have been on diets, eating plans, and diet supplements. I tried them all, repeatedly, but *"the flesh profits nothing."* I was left with no long-term change, no real profit (benefit).

 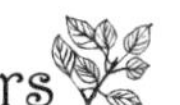

Then I began to take the words of Jesus seriously. Jesus said that they were *"spirit, and...life."* The apostle Paul called them *"weapons"* in 2 Corinthians 10:4: *"The weapons of our warfare are not carnal."* Most overweight people have experienced the frustration of fighting this spiritual battle with carnal or fleshly weapons. Dieting is a carnal weapon. Crash dieting starves your body, but it does not affect the spirit of overeating that is inside. That is why you can go on a diet and lose weight, then stop the diet and gain it all back. *Jesus never put a glutton on a diet.* A person can be just as obsessed with food when he is on a diet as when he is overeating. He still thinks about food just as much.

There are some highly successful diet plans that allow you to eat a great deal of food, but only certain types. You can have some things in unlimited amounts, such as carrot sticks and celery. Instead of eating potato chips and cookies, you munch on carrots and celery. Instead of eating huge servings of baked beans and potato salad, you eat huge servings of green beans and baked fish.

It is like a heroin addict going on methadone—the addiction is still there, but you take a substitute instead of the more destructive drug. The glutton continues in gluttony but eats low-calorie foods instead of high-calorie foods. And he loses weight. *The urge to overeat is still there. The habit of overeating is still there.*

When a person eventually grows tired of preparing special diet foods and considering everything he must eat for the diet, he eventually goes back to foods he ate before the diet. Because he has not dealt with his gluttony, he regains the lost weight. But Jesus said, *"Therefore if the Son makes you free, **you shall be free indeed**"* (John 8:36, emphasis added).

Freedom from Restrictions

Being free means not having to bring special food with you to a restaurant. Being free is not spending half your day planning menus. Being free is not cooking one meal for your family and a separate meal for yourself. Being free is not having to pass up half the food your hostess serves. Being free is being free indeed.

When you are on a diet, you lose weight. When you stop the diet, you regain the weight. It's like a roller coaster, with each period of gaining more discouraging than the last. Some people eventually give up. Their weight increases, out of control, leading to many serious health complications. Weight climbs past 200 to 300, 350, or even 400 pounds. I have known women who eventually weighed over 500 pounds. At that point, your freedom is almost non-existent!

Even being 20 percent overweight makes a person 50 percent more likely to develop high blood pressure and twice as likely to develop heart disease. Obesity is found in 85 percent of adult onset diabetes. It significantly increases the risk of breast cancer, arterial disease, and pregnancy complications. Overweight people are less likely to survive surgery. Their very life expectancy is shortened.

Jesus said, *"The thief does not come except to steal, and to kill, and to destroy"* (John 10:10). The bondage of food addiction does steal, kill, and destroy.

But then Jesus said the wonderful news, *"I have come that they may have life, and that they may have it more abundantly"* (v. 10). Jesus came to set *you* free, to give you life, and that life is abundant life. Freedom is awesome and *possible.*

Power for Freedom

Your pastor may or may not talk about eating disorders, but the Bible certainly does. Scripture speaks eloquently about the inward struggles, the discouraging failures, and the secret eating. Sadly, many pastors are hesitant to speak openly for fear of offending. Many of them have never been under the bondage of a compulsive behavior, so they don't understand the real bondage it creates. A woman told me that when she sought help in her church, people told her that size "didn't really matter," even though she weighed over 350 pounds! Her body was literally being destroyed, her soul and spirit were in condemnation, and Christians told her, "It doesn't really matter."

I don't believe I have ever heard a person tell someone with a drinking or drug problem that "it really doesn't matter" how much he drinks or how many drugs he takes. We are afraid to "hurt someone's feelings" if he is a glutton. Let me tell you from experience, *that person is already hurting more than you can imagine.*

The Bible is not so silent on the subject. *"The drunkard and the glutton will come to poverty"* (Proverbs 23:21). Again, in Proverbs 23:2, *"Put a knife to your throat if you are a man given to appetite"* (put the sword of God's Word to your throat if you are a person given to appetite). In Philippians 3:18–19, Paul told us,

> *For many walk, of whom I have told you often, and now tell you even weeping, that they are the enemies of the cross of Christ: whose end is destruction, whose god is their belly.*

A glutton or binge eater is not as easy on himself as some of his church-going friends might believe. He knows what he is dealing with. A questionnaire given to a number of overweight people asked the question, "Do you believe that it is sinful to overeat?" The unanimous answer was, *"Yes!"*

I was desperately aware that what I was doing was wrong, but I didn't know how to get out of it. I was my biggest critic! Inwardly, my thoughts were like those of David in Psalm 51:3: *"For I acknowledge my transgressions, and my sin is always before me."* One look in the mirror confirmed my weakness, but the Bible is filled with wonderful words of hope for overeaters.

The "job description" of the Holy Spirit given in Isaiah 61:1 is to *"preach good tidings"* (give real hope) and to *"heal the brokenhearted"* (God sees our tears of frustration and sorrow over our inability to control our eating). Verse one also says that the anointing of the Lord is sent to *"proclaim liberty to*

the captives" (you can be free for the rest of your life) and the *"opening of the prison to those who are bound"* (God wants you to be released—He has opened the prison door). That image of imprisonment certainly describes the inward bondage of the one unsuccessfully battling any addiction—to food, alcohol, drugs, sexual perversion—brokenhearted, captive, in prison, and bound up.

Chapter 3
Seeds of Gluttony

People often ask me, "Diane, when did you *know* you were truly healed of gluttony?" I have to answer honestly that, for the whole first year, I had to keep pinching myself to believe it was going to last. After many years of frustration, disappointment, and dead-end diets, I knew it would take a miracle to set me free!

I did not thoroughly understand that I could be completely healed of this eating disorder and be free for the rest of my life. I was hoping for the ability to keep my eating under control. But *"eye has not seen, nor ear heard, nor have entered into the heart of man the things which God has prepared for those who love Him"* (1 Corinthians 2:9).

Many times I dreamed I would be thin, free, and "normal." Yet I always woke up to the same driving desire to eat. I had a constant obsession with food. Now, for the first time, it was gone—not under control, but gone! Depression and self-hatred were lifted from me as giant weights never to return. After years and years of constant weight changes, I had the extraordinary experience of being able to wear the same clothes year after year.

Every change of season was a new reminder that I was free!

Help for Your Problem

When one of our daughters was growing up, sometimes life seemed to overwhelm her. Unable to protect her from all the pains of life, I would hold her in my arms, pat her back, and tell her, "It's going to be all right. Everything is going to be okay. You are going to have a wonderful life." For many years she would come to me in difficult times and say, "Mom, would you hug me and tell me everything's going to be all right?" That is a lot of what ministry is—just assuring others that God is going to bring them through.

For all of you who have struggled so long and hard with compulsive eating, you who feel discouraged and overwhelmed, if Jesus could be there with you in His flesh, I know He would do the same for you. He would wrap His big, strong arms around you and tell you, "It's going to be all right. I can help you. I know the answer, and you can be free."

How Does Gluttony Begin?

To understand the solution, we need to have some understanding of how gluttony begins in a life, how it becomes a stronghold. Knowing the truth is part of what sets us free. We have a number of scriptural examples of Jesus providing food to nourish people's physical bodies. There was always a consistent order. First spirits were fed; then bodies were fed. First He taught and ministered to the spirit; then He multiplied the loaves and fishes to feed the body.

> *And they said to Him, "We have here only five loaves and two fish." He said, "Bring them here to Me." Then He commanded the multitudes to sit down on the grass. And He took the five loaves and the two fish, and looking up to heaven, He blessed and broke and gave the loaves to the disciples; and the disciples gave to the multitudes. So they all ate and were filled, and they took up twelve baskets full of the fragments that remained.*
>
> (Matthew 14:17–20)

Gluttony begins when this system gets out of order. A person feels frustrated, bored, angry, or lonely; but rather than dealing with the spiritual problem, he eats. These are examples of the *"deceptive food"* spoken of in Proverbs 23:3. It is food eaten for the wrong reason—to avoid dealing with the deeper problem.

Loving Jesus First

Jesus said that one commandment is the greatest and the most important; it is foundational. Here it is.

> *"You shall love the* Lord *your God with all your heart, with all your soul, with all your mind, and*

> *with all your strength." This is the first commandment.* (Mark 12:30)

In gluttony, at some point, a person begins to eat when he is frustrated, worried, angry, sad, lonely, or bored. Rather than turning to God for comfort and help, he turns to food. That is why Paul said in Philippians 3:19 that a glutton's *"god is* [his] *belly."*

Spiritual Seed

When we eat this way, the seeds of gluttony are sown. We are told in Galatians 6:7–8,

> *Do not be deceived, God is not mocked; for whatever a man sows, that he will also reap. For he who sows to his flesh* [eating for the wrong reasons] *will of the flesh reap corruption* [gluttony], *but he who sows to the Spirit* [seeking help in God's Word] *will of the Spirit reap everlasting life* [a Spirit-controlled life].

A person who has never eaten out of frustration, anger, boredom, or loneliness finds it hard to imagine why a person would do this. But, *as with all sin, in the beginning, one finds real pleasure in overeating.* As a drunk drinks himself into a stupor, a glutton eats himself into a stupor. The food tastes good and seems to help him forget about his problems. Unfortunately, as with all sin, when the pleasure begins to wear off, the addictive quality of sin does not. Jesus warns us, *"Whoever commits sin is a slave of sin"* (John 8:34).

Seeking Solace in Wrong Places

The basic problems that caused the person to seek solace in food in the first place have not been dealt with. As a result, the problems are only increased. More often than not, depression accompanies gluttony. The original frustration is accompanied by even greater frustration as the eating gets out of control. The original anger is accompanied by condemnation and greater anger at oneself. "I hate myself when I overeat like this" is a common response.

Tears of anger, frustration, and hopelessness accompany each binge. It is not unlike drug addiction in that the "highs" become less high, and the "lows" become more and more unbearable. Proverbs says, *"Bread gained by deceit is sweet to a man, but afterward his mouth will be filled with gravel"* (Proverbs 20:17).

Anger and Your Soul

I receive letters from all over the world from men and women who have read this book and received healing and all the weight loss that goes with it. I recently received this letter from a woman in Australia:

"For five years now I had been battling with a stronghold of food addiction. I got the book, couldn't put it down, and was instantly free. Four months down the track, I am back down to 52 kilograms

[115 pounds] and still losing weight. My coeliac is cured [a disease she had suffered with]. My food tastes great, and I feel free indeed. You gave me the secrets and I thank you and God daily."

We all love testimonies like that, but here is a very different letter I received. From the first words, the tone was hostile and bitter.

"I bought your book and I read it. I followed it for two weeks—*to the letter.* [She underlined that part!] It didn't work. I also went to [a Bible-based weight loss group]. I won't be going back there! Do you have something else that could help me?"

Actually, I think I could help her, but I would begin by looking at something I don't believe she even sees. I believe it is very possible that this woman's healing is being blocked by unresolved anger.

Anger can play a huge part in food addictions. It is obvious that this woman is a Christian from the places she was looking to for help.

Unfortunately, many Christians do not believe that they can be a Christian and still experience anger. Sometimes people wrongly believe that anger and sin are the same thing. The Bible suggests otherwise.

Anger is not something that is covered up in the Scriptures at all. There are over five hundred references to anger and wrath in the Bible. It speaks plainly of the Lord God's anger and of Jesus' anger on several occasions; in the book of Ephesians, Paul said, *"Be angry, and do not sin"* (Ephesians 4:26). It is the way that anger is expressed that can become sinful.

Many, many verses warn us against certain ways of expressing our anger. Anger can be directed in many destructive ways toward ourselves and others. Angry words that belittle and humiliate another person are terrible, and terribly wrong. Jesus condemned them in the strongest possible terms: *"Whoever says, 'You fool!' shall be in danger of hell fire"* (Matthew 5:22).

Physical violence is a destructive way to express anger. We all know the wrong ways to express anger. What many Christians aren't so aware of are the healthy ways to express anger. Anger can bring about positive changes in our world. For example, someone can feel so angry about people driving after they have been drinking that he seeks to bring about a change in order to save lives.

The ability to appropriately express anger in marriage is necessary to keep relationships in balance. One time my husband and I were in a disagreement about something. We had the kind of quarrel that every married couple has from time to time. I didn't feel that he was listening to what I was trying to say, so I was feeling angry.

He said, "Are you mad at me now?" I said, very coldly, "No, I am not mad." That was a lie. I was feeling very angry.

Holding that anger in and not expressing it in a healthy way was wrong. If I had continued not to express my anger, I could have been in danger of giving a *"foothold to the devil"* (Ephesians 4:27 TLB). We are warned about letting the sun go down on our anger (see Ephesians 4:26), holding it in until it becomes a bitter thing and begins to poison our lives and words and thoughts.

Finally I said, "I am angry. I am angry that you didn't listen to what I was saying." That was not a sinful expression of anger. An appropriate expression of anger allows us to continue to be *"kind…* [and] *tenderhearted, forgiving one another"* (v. 32).

Anger toward God

Of all the unresolved anger, the most destructive is anger toward God. The Bible doesn't hide this type of anger either.

"The Lord respected Abel and his offering, but He did not respect Cain and his offering. And Cain was very angry" (Genesis 4:4–5). Cain was so angry with God for not accepting his offering that he eventually killed his brother, Abel.

God's response to our anger is quite different from what some might expect. He did not strike Cain with a lightening bolt. He began to ask Cain some questions that would have caused Cain to understand why his offering had been unacceptable. God said, *"If you do well, will you not be accepted* [just as Abel was]?" (v. 7).

When the Pharisees became angry because Jesus healed on the Sabbath day, Jesus' response was just like His Father's response to Cain; it was a question. *"Are you angry with Me because I made a man completely well on the Sabbath?"* (John 7:23). When God observes anger toward Him, it seems

He often begins to question the inner motivations in a way that could really help.

Things can happen that seem unfair and unjust, and God can wind up with the blame.

Are you angry inside? Do you even understand why? I believe that God can help you resolve those awful, hateful feelings when you come to Him in honesty. You might begin with, "God, I feel a lot of anger inside, and I'm not even sure who I am angry at. I may even be angry at You; but whatever it is, I want to live in the freedom You made possible. Would You help me?"

I believe He will. I believe that kind of honesty and humility is very powerful. I think that is part of what Jesus meant when He said, *"Blessed are the meek* [humble], *for they shall inherit the earth"* (Matthew 5:5). Freedom from addictions is part of your inheritance in God. Don't let anger or unforgiveness block your healing.

The Beginning of the End of Gluttony

Because gluttony begins in the spirit, the solution also begins in the spirit. It began by sowing to the flesh, and it will end by sowing to the Spirit!

In the past I had sown to the flesh by eating during my times of depression, frustration, boredom, and guilt. Now I began to sow to the Spirit by literally making a decision to make my battle spiritual. This might be by fasting, changing my activity, changing my location, or changing my attitude. In each case, it was making my *faith* an action. God, who knows the secret motivation of every act, receives it as spiritual seed. Becoming focused on God gives us a single-minded vision. This is how you can sow to the Spirit.

Every glutton has experienced the almost "supernatural" urge to overeat, even eating things they don't really like. The eating is unreasonable, unnatural, and unrelenting in its desire. Proverbs 27:7 tells us that to the full soul, even a honeycomb isn't tempting, *"but to a hungry soul every bitter thing is sweet."* In other words, there is a type of eating that originates from "soul hunger," not body hunger. Obviously, you cannot fill an empty soul with hamburgers and french fries. When you swallow food, there is not some "soul-esophagus" that takes the food into your soul. Now as ridiculous as that may sound, this is what many people are attempting to do. Physical food is taken in to fill a spiritual or emotional need.

Jesus gives an invitation that speaks directly to this soul pain, which is part of life. He says,

> *Come to Me, all you who labor and are heavy laden, and I will give you rest. Take My yoke upon you and learn from Me, for I am gentle and lowly in heart, and* ***you will find rest for your souls****. For My yoke is easy and My burden is light.*
> (Matthew 11:28–30, emphasis added)

He is speaking of and acknowledging that emotional part of us. *"Heavy laden"* means frustrated, worried, lonely, sad, or angry. Everyone relates to this description emotionally.

Jesus didn't mean to bring Him our heavy grocery bags. He is speaking of the kind of inward stuff that weighs us down inside and creates a "soul vacuum" that must be filled, one way or another.

Soul hunger cannot be satisfied with food or any other fleshly sustenance. No matter how much you eat, you are not satisfied. You go to bed stuffed with food but with no satisfaction or rest for that soul hunger.

In Matthew 11:28–29, Jesus made a promise that can be counted on. He said that we would find *"rest for* [our] *souls."* He did not say that He would bring us rest for our souls on a silver platter. We are to *"come"* and to *"take,"* and then "[we] *will find rest for* [our] *souls."*

Let's apply this specifically to that hunger that originates in the soul. How do we *"come to"* Jesus in times of distress? We have to make choices.

The first choice is to *"come." This means that we make a spiritual intervention in our physical world.* We literally change what we are doing in order to *"come to"* Him. We don't try to solve our pain or place a blame for it. We don't beat ourselves up emotionally. We *"come to"* Him.

Second, we "take His yoke." We become inwardly and outwardly obedient to our understanding of what Jesus would do.

Here is an example of how this brings healing. Let's say that Mary has had a "bad day." She has come home frustrated and angry at herself. Something unfair happened, and she really blew it. She feels a heavy burden inside and find herself in front of the refrigerator. She looks in and grabs something handy. Then she picks up the phone (all this time she is inwardly feeling a great soul hunger). She talks to one of her friends, who winds up saying some things about some other people that Mary didn't really feel good about. She hangs up and now she is really feeling bad. Unconsciously, she flips on the television to try to cover up what she is feeling inside. She heads back to the refrigerator. Before long, she is caught in a cycle of eating that she will deeply regret and not really understand.

Now, let's allow Mary to make a spiritual intervention by making some right choices at this critical point. Mary still comes home having had a "bad day." She is frustrated and angry at herself. She again finds herself in front of the refrigerator when she remembers His words, *"Come to Me"* (Matthew 11:28). Mary realizes that she is in a vulnerable place emotionally. She physically removes herself from the present temptation. Perhaps she goes on a quick walk; perhaps she goes to a room where she can shut the door—the logistics are not nearly as important as the decision she made to *"come to"* Him.

Almost as soon as she gets alone with Jesus, she begins to pour out her heart. She can be honest with Him. She can be angry and hurt and frustrated. Then she says, "Lord, I'm sorry. Will You forgive me?"

He might answer back, "Of course I will, but do you know what you need to do?" Mary remembers several people and incidents that she is still angry over. Jesus said, *"Take My yoke"* (Matthew 11:29). When Mary makes the decision to forgive those who have willfully wronged her or hurt her, she is "taking His yoke." Her soul is brought into a position of rest. She can now go back into her day, and the outcome will be completely different. She can still talk to her friend, still go to the refrigerator to begin dinner, but her soul is okay.

She has "sown to the Spirit," and she has "reaped from the Spirit."

Similar scenarios are played out in our lives in a thousand different ways. There is always a place of decision. The Bible calls it the *"way of escape"* in 1 Corinthians 10:13. It is *always* there.

As I began to see my battle as spiritual, I began to win it. The condemnation that Satan heaped on me was losing its power over me. That urge to eat to my destruction began to subside.

First comes the inner healing; then comes the outer healing that is the weight loss. After the inner healing, *that awful, constant, nagging urge to overeat is gone.* When I dieted as a glutton, I was confronted with temptation from the moment I woke up in the morning. I didn't have to stand against eating a few times a day; I had to stand against eating every fifteen minutes! Cutting back on eating is such a simple thing now.

Where to Begin

In Matthew 17:20–21, Jesus tells us,

> *If you have faith as a mustard seed, you will say to this mountain, "Move from here to there," and it will move; and nothing will be impossible for you. However, this kind does not go out except by prayer and fasting.*

Gluttony is one of those difficult kinds of strongholds. There is sometimes a lifetime pattern of overeating that must be broken. Eating carrot sticks and celery, instead of potato chips and cookies, does not break this pattern.

No one became a glutton or compulsive eater in one day. Gluttony becomes a stronghold because, as Jesus said, *"Whoever commits sin is a slave of sin"* (John 8:34). It did not begin as a stronghold. It began as a small seed, and it started to grow when we first began to "sow to the flesh" by eating from frustration, loneliness, anger, self-condemnation, and habit.

Each time we used food in this way, this urge to indulge grew a little bigger and a little stronger. Gluttony consists of two forces. One is an overwhelming desire to eat, with constant, nagging thoughts of food. This is the spiritual part that we call the "spirit of overeating." The other part is simply habit. A compulsive eater often gets to the point where he is actually unaware of some of the food he eats. Overeating has become as natural as breathing.

Hidden Sin

One woman told me how God showed her that she always scooped a heaping spoonful of peanut butter for herself when she made her children peanut butter sandwiches. She said she was honestly unaware of eating the peanut butter.

Eventually gluttony, or the spirit of overeating, becomes like a strong, hardy, living plant inside us. It is a stronghold, a fortified place surrounded by excuses, self-deception, and habits that can be formed over a lifetime. Each time we choose God over our eating, we chip away another root of the stronghold.

Gluttony is like a huge tree that can be blown over by a mild wind when the root structure is destroyed. The spirit of overeating shrivels up a little more with each victory until it finally dies. Gluttony begins with sowing to the flesh. It will end by sowing to the Spirit, in faith.

Daily Fasting

God's Word says,

> *Whatever a man sows, that he will also reap. For he who sows to his flesh* [eating out of frustration, boredom, anger, or other reasons] *will of the flesh reap corruption* [gluttony, compulsive eating, obsession with food], *but he who sows to the Spirit* [daily periods of fasting] *will of the Spirit reap everlasting life* [a Spirit-controlled life]. (Galatians 6:7–9)

Seeds are tiny things and yet they carry life in them. God chose a Seed to redeem the human race. If God chose it, then we can see that seeds are very, very powerful. The Bible is filled with references to seeds. Jesus spoke of seeds over and over. *"If you have faith* ***as a mustard seed****"* (Matthew 17:20, emphasis added). *"The kingdom of heaven is* ***like a mustard seed****"* (Matthew 13:31, emphasis added).

When Jesus said to *"love your enemies, bless those who curse you, do good to those who hate you, and pray for those who spitefully use you and persecute you"* (Matthew 5:44), He was telling us to be proactive in our response to evil. Sow love, sow blessing—that is what God does. We increase the good in the earth when we imitate God in this way, and we increase the good in our lives when we consciously sow good seeds in them.

A seed must be sown in faith. That is just as true of a natural seed as it is of a spiritual seed. You don't plant and water a seed unless you *believe* in that seed and the power that is contained in it. Seeds are good things to believe in! They produce what they promise they will produce. By that I mean human seeds produce humans. Tomato seeds produce tomatoes. Wheat seeds produce wheat.

Your faith in seeds will determine how you approach your eating. It will produce the outcome.

Jesus said, *"If you have faith as a mustard seed..."* (Matthew 17:20). Evidently, small seeds can produce huge harvests in God. To put it another way, if you win the small battles, God will make sure you will win the big ones.

Fasting before God

My approach to weight loss was always to "diet before men." Jesus said that when we fast we are to *"fast...to your Father who is in the secret place; and your Father who sees in secret will reward you openly"* (Matthew 6:16, 18). He did not say, "If you fast," but rather, *"When you fast"* (v. 16). If you need control with your eating, you can sow control with your eating.

This fasting should be at a level that you can do. To bring an offering to God is a serious, holy thing. Perhaps one hour is all you can do in the beginning, but that one hour, when offered to God, becomes a spiritual seed.

If you look at the one hour with your natural mind, it looks ridiculous to expect it to begin to change your life, but it will. God redeemed the entire human race with one Seed, His Son Jesus. He can certainly heal your addiction—no matter what it is—with small seeds of obedience.

Jesus said, *"If anyone wants to do His will, he shall know concerning the doctrine, whether it is from God"* (John 7:17). I love doing what Jesus said to do in different life situations. You truly experience the secret of it only by doing it. Everything Jesus said is important because He was God speaking things that had been hidden from the beginning of time, and His words were *"spirit"* (John 6:63). Each statement about how we are to live is pure gold; there is a great, unexpected treasure in it that we can understand only when we do it.

Let me give you an example of what I mean. Many years ago, I had an enemy. This person was doing me great harm and seemed to have the power to influence a number of people against me. The more I tried to defend myself, the more difficult the situation became. I was becoming bitter and angry.

I finally got out my Bible and began to read Matthew 5:44: *"Bless those who curse you, do good to those who hate you, and pray for those who spitefully use you."* Yuck! I certainly did not want to love or pray for or bless this person, but there was no getting around it, and everything I was doing was bringing only more failure and pain. (Sound familiar?)

Grudgingly at first, I began to do the will of the Father, just as Jesus said. Now, nothing in the situation had changed except this one thing—I had secretly made a spiritual intervention into my physical world by doing what Jesus said.

I had no understanding of how it could help. I had no idea what effect it would have. I was just hoping that it would help me to forgive and be freed from the awful bitterness.

The most amazing thing happened. From the moment I began this secret obedience, this person began to lose the ability to influence people against me. It was as if I had a secret defender. Remember what Jesus said about His words being *"spirit"* (John 6:63). They were! They had a spiritual power when implemented in my life through obedience.

Eventually, my enemy became my friend, but I will never forget how much I learned about praying for enemies. There was this "treasure" hidden inside obedience. It was only when I began to do His will that I knew the truth of it.

Spiritual Interventions

Spiritual intervention is when a person deliberately changes his or her physical circumstances for a spiritual purpose. Tithing would be a good example of spiritual intervention. The Bible makes some wonderful promises to tithers in Malachi 3:10–12. God says,

> *"Bring all the tithes into the storehouse, that there may be food in My house, and try Me now in this," says the* Lord *of hosts, "If I will not open for you the windows of heaven and pour out for you such blessing that there will not be room enough to receive it. And I will rebuke the devourer for your sakes, so that he will not destroy the fruit of your ground, nor shall the vine fail to bear fruit for you in the field."*

That is in the Bible. It lies there inactive until a person makes a spiritual intervention. The person deliberately changes his physical circumstances for a spiritual purpose. He deliberately decreases his financial resources by writing a check or laying aside cash for a spiritual purpose (to be obedient in tithing); and as he gives that money into his church offering, he has made a spiritual intervention. That word from Malachi now has been activated by the individual's deliberate act of obedience.

Anyone who has tithed understands the unusual blessing and protection that God has provided for us through the tithe, but it is activated only by doing it.

This is why these periods of fasting, even for what seem like insignificant amounts of time in the beginning, contain within them a power that is released only by doing it. It becomes spiritual seed. I could tell you over and over, but you won't understand until you do it. God adds to it something unique to your individual situation that so increases you inwardly that you are changed inside. Something at the very root of the problem begins to change.

This type of fasting actually attacks gluttony at both the physical and spiritual levels. Releasing your faith to God as you sow control attacks the spiritual force of gluttony. The physical side of fasting helps to break the habit. There is a saying, "Sow an action, and you reap a habit."

My healing began when I literally applied this Scripture to my compulsive eating and released my faith to God for a miracle! During my healing, not even my husband knew I was fasting. My diets had always been obvious—one meal for him, something else for me. Now I would eat breakfast and fast until dinner. When he came home, I ate regular meals with him, but smaller portions.

This fasting was not just another way of losing weight. It was a secret commitment between God and me. Every time I passed up some food, I released my faith to God for healing. This is where the *power* is. The apostle John said, *"As many as received Him* [chose Him], *to them He gave the right* [*"power,"* KJV] *to become children of God"* (John 1:12). We don't have to provide the power, just the will. To this day, I am not a person strong in willpower, but I have learned the strength of leaning on the power of Jesus Christ.

Secrets to Effective Fasting

Be faithful. Be faithful. Be faithful. One hour of faithfulness is much more important than a plan to fast all day that doesn't happen. This fasting should not be a week-long fast or a three-day fast, but rather a daily period of fasting. Eventually, skipping one meal a day is an ideal and scripturally sound way of fasting. (See Chapter 4.)

In the beginning your body will experience hunger—real, physical hunger. It may be the first time in a long, long time that it has experienced actual hunger. You may think, "I'm going to starve without food because I missed a meal!!" Satan, the deceiver, may try to pull you away from God's Word by planting discouraging thoughts. He will try to tell you it isn't going to work. "You have always been overweight, and you always will be overweight." He will try to get you to binge. But Scripture says, *"Resist the devil and he will flee from you"* (James 4:7).

David wrote in Psalm 25:1–2, *"To You, O LORD, I lift up my soul. O my God, I trust in You; let me not be ashamed; let not my enemies triumph over me."*

When you open your eyes in the morning, let these thoughts be in your heart and mind. Purpose in your heart each morning which seed you are going to sow. Remember, it is better to start small and stay faithful. It is very important to your own spiritual life to keep your word to God.

Don't wait until lunchtime to decide you are going to fast lunch! One woman said she purposed to fast until noon. At noon she found she could go longer, so she determined to go until 2:00 PM. At 2:00 she found she could fast longer, so she decided to fast until dinner. And she did.

Proverb 3:3 talks about writing on the *"tablet of your heart."* I found that if I resolved to fast a certain time before the Lord, I never failed. If I only thought, "Maybe I will sow some fasting today," I usually didn't make it.

Does God Mean More to You?

I used to wonder why God would have us fast. Fasting has a way of helping us focus on God. It is a great strengthening tool for our inner man. When I am fasting before God, and I am tempted to eat, I simply ask myself, "Which means more to me? This food or Jesus?" Looking at food this way makes it easy for me to choose. I love the Lord with all my heart, and suddenly that food doesn't mean much.

Sometimes people have problem foods. By that I mean that a particular food is especially tempting to you. It is a specific food that you consistently tend to overeat. It might be ice cream for some, chocolate or potato chips for others. Whatever it is, you can actually take the food in your hands and make an out-loud statement that you love God more than that food. Say, "Lord, I love You more than ice cream." Put it back in the freezer. The next time you are tempted, take it out again and say, "Lord, I love You more than ice cream." Unusual things will happen in your attitude toward that "irresistible" food product.

Your choice can be reinforced when you pass by that food the next time you go to the supermarket. Gumdrops were one of those foods for me. During the time of my healing, I chose not to have them in the house. It was a temporary thing. Now, I have a jar of gumdrops on my desk all the time. Each time I see it, it is a reminder of what God did in my life. The jar goes down very slowly because it is just a jar of gumdrops now. It has lost its power in my life.

Sowing Good Seed

In 2 Corinthians 9:6 we are told, *"He who sows sparingly will also reap sparingly, and he who sows bountifully will also reap bountifully."* What is frugal sowing, and what is bountiful sowing, with regard to our fasting? We are told, *"The Lord does not see as man sees; for man looks at the outward appearance, but the Lord looks at the heart"* (1 Samuel 16:7). God is always looking at our hearts.

Jesus was greatly moved by a certain type of giving. Remember the little widow that Jesus commended in Mark 12:44? It was because she gave *"of her want"* (KJV) that Jesus commended her. He wasn't impressed with the rich people who *"put in out of their abundance,"* but oh, how He noticed the widow! How He felt her faith reach out to God as she gave *"all that she had."* Jesus was moved by this bountiful giving. She made a spiritual intervention by her giving. She deliberately changed her physical circumstances for a spiritual purpose, and Jesus noticed it.

Results of Sparse Sowing

Contrast this with frugal giving. If you normally do not eat breakfast, then not eating breakfast is not "giving of your want." It is not bountiful giving, and it is not sowing from your heart.

A woman I know actually did this! She didn't seem to be having much success, yet she said, "I've been fasting a meal every day!" I asked her which meal she was fasting, and she said breakfast (the smallest meal). I asked her if she normally ate breakfast, since most overweight people don't.

"Well, no," was her reply. She sowed sparingly and was reaping sparingly! God knew she didn't eat breakfast! Even if she did, this would be the smallest and least significant meal to fast. He was looking for a heart response that said, "Lord, I love You more than this food." He was looking for a heart that soared in faith as it gave in joy! Instead, He found deception and avarice.

Jesus said in Mark 10:29 that it is only what we give up *"for* [His] *sake and the gospel's"* that will be returned to us a hundredfold. God looks for our inner motivation.

Sowing Bountifully

If your boss tells you that you *must* work through your lunch hour, then not eating lunch is not sowing bountifully. If you gave up lunch because your boss said you *must,* it was not for the sake of Jesus. However, sometimes working through your lunch hour is bountiful giving. Perhaps you resolved in your heart that morning that you were going to fast lunch. God might have arranged for your boss to ask you to work through your lunch hour to help you make it. Man looks at the outward appearance, but God looks at the heart, the inner motivation.

Not only does God look at the inner motivation (or heart) but He, of course, also correctly measures the love and sacrifice and faith that is represented. Again, He correctly measured the widow's mite as more than the rich man's large gift.

The Bible says that the *"steps of a good man are ordered by the Lord"* (Psalm 37:23). Expect God to get involved when you sow in faith! Many times when I decided to fast, God brought activities into my day that made it almost impossible for me to find time to eat. He made it easy for me.

It is the motivation of our hearts and giving in faith that determines bountiful giving. Sometimes not eating one cookie is bountiful giving! God sees that one cookie in the same way He saw the widow's mite.

If you have the most trouble with overeating at bedtime, this is the time you should fast before God. This would be giving from your want. If you have trouble because you eat while fixing dinner for your family, this is the time you should fast before God. If you do not eat all the time, but eat too much when you do eat, begin by cutting out second helpings and offering the sacrifice to God.

Whenever you are overeating is the time to sow from your want. That is loving God with all your strength in regard to eating.

One Day at a Time

Jesus told us to take one day at a time. *"Therefore do not worry about tomorrow, for tomorrow will worry about its own things. Sufficient for the day is its own trouble"* (Matthew 6:34). Jesus is telling us not to try to handle the whole problem at once. We have enough grace to walk in total victory for each day; but if we focus on the 50 or 100 pounds we have to lose, we aren't going to reach our goal.

I remember getting up in the morning and weighing myself. Seeing how much weight I needed to lose was such a discouragement that, instead of beginning small, I thought about all the food I was going to have to do without. I would consider how long it would take, and often I would give up before I began!

Humanly, we always look at the whole problem, and it seems impossible. But Jesus taught us to start small and have faith in God. He said, *"The things which are impossible with men are possible with God"* (Luke 18:27). A number of years ago, a man lost over 150 pounds after reading this book. Now, that seems impossible to me, but he did it with God, and you can, too. How often he must have felt that his situation was so discouraging that he wanted to just give up.

We become like the fishermen in Luke 5 who were fishing all night. Jesus said, *"Let down your nets for a catch"* (v. 4). The fishermen answered, *"Master, we have toiled all night"* (v. 5). They were thinking that they had cast the net over and over, and it would be useless to cast the net one more time. We often think, "But I've tried every diet, and nothing has worked. What good will it do to stop between-meal eating or to try to change my activities?"

When the fishermen cast their nets at the word of Jesus, they caught more fish than they could handle! Jesus is also involved in *our* lives. We are not just fasting between meals; we are sowing our fast to God as a farmer sows seed. We are each watching eagerly for a harvest. That man who lost 150 pounds had his miracle harvest!

Faithful Living

I found that as I tried to be faithful for just that day, for that hour, the weeks took care of themselves. How much emotional illness is a result of anxiety about the future or guilt over the past! The God who created us tells us that worry and guilt will overload our circuits! *"Do not worry about tomorrow.…Sufficient for the day is its own trouble"* (Matthew 6:34). Just try to make it this day.

Jesus told us, *"He who is faithful in what is least* [daily periods of fasting] *is faithful also in much* [total weight loss]" (Luke 16:10). The more faithful I was in the small decisions, the more faithful I was in the big ones.

Our Free-Will Choice

No one can sow the seed but you. No one else can do it for you. The choice is yours. You never lose your free will as far as God is concerned. You can try to blame others for your choices. You may blame your husband. "He makes me so mad, I can't keep from eating!" You may blame your family. "I came from a fat family." Or your childhood eating habits may have been poor. "I was raised to eat wrong." You may blame the devil. "Satan simply has me under his thumb with my eating."

God tells us the choice is ours. *"I have set before you life and death, blessing and cursing; therefore choose life"* (Deuteronomy 30:19).

> *Do you not know that to whom you present yourselves slaves* [whom you choose] *to obey, you are that one's slaves whom you obey, whether of sin leading to death, or of obedience leading to righteousness?* (Romans 6:16)

God will supply the power, but we must supply the will.

There was a time in my life when it was impossible for me to control my eating for any length of time. But *"the things which are impossible with men are possible with God"* (Luke 18:27).

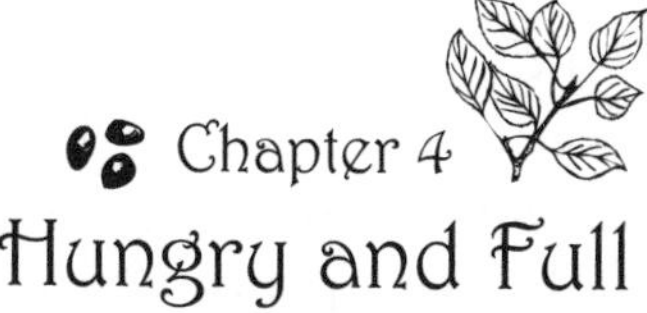

Chapter 4
Hungry and Full

The book of Genesis is a good reference for beginning to understand how God intended our relationship with food to be. We hear a lot of messages about food. We hear a lot of "shoulds" and "should nots," but what was God's plan from the beginning?

> *In the beginning God created the heavens and the earth....Then God said, "Let Us make man in Our image."...The* Lord *God planted a garden eastward in Eden, and there He put the man whom He had formed....And the* Lord *God commanded the man, saying, "Of every tree of the garden you may freely eat."...Then God saw everything that He had made, and indeed it was very good.*
>
> (Genesis 1:1, 26; 2:8, 16; 1:31)

In this man whom God created, He put a response called "hunger." This response came when the man needed food. The system was very good. And God put another response in the man called "full." This response came when his body had enough food. It was also very good. These responses, hungry and full, calculated exactly how much food the man needed to eat, for he was *"fearfully and wonderfully made"* (Psalm 139:14).

Some foods were heavy, and this full response came quickly and lasted a long time. Some foods were lighter, and the full response came slower. But no matter what was eaten—bananas or blueberries—these two responses were his guides for eating and not eating. There were no gluttons in the Garden.

Recapturing Your Natural Responses

When a newborn baby is brought home from the hospital, he makes good use of these responses. He cries when he is hungry, and we feed him. When he is full he stops eating, and we stop trying to feed him. It all works very well—just as God intended. We are born with these responses, so we don't have to learn them. Doctors have even given this instinctive action a name. It is called "demand feeding." Babies eat when they are hungry and stop eating when they are full.

Unfortunately, this is usually the last we hear of these hungry and full responses. A child still responds to these God-given responses, and we see how well it works. One rarely sees an overweight child. But as he grows, we begin to give the child a cracker when he is bored or a cookie when he is tired. By the time the child is five years old, if he sits down to dinner and is not hungry, he is often told, "You can just sit right there until you clean your plate."

If the child cleans his plate, he is told he is a "good boy." If the child does not clean his plate, he is told he is "bad."

Reasons for Eating

We learn to eat because "it's time," "you'll feel better if you eat," "you *might* get hungry," "people are starving in India," or "you will hurt Aunt Mabel's feelings if you don't eat." These are all typical reasons for eating. We are also continually bombarded with articles on dieting. Food fads are a part of the American way of life. Certain types of eating gain wide approval and are "preached as the gospel" by their adherents. Eating becomes complicated, confusing, and guilt-producing to many people.

By adulthood these God-given responses of hungry and full have often been hidden so successfully that many count calories, carbohydrates, fats, or whatever to determine how much food they need. *Many never dream of skipping a meal just because they aren't hungry.* At best, we simply don't eat quite as much.

Don't Eat Anything If You Aren't Hungry

One of the first things God showed me about my eating was to *eat only when I was hungry.* Don't eat anything unless you are really hungry.

That thought was so new to me that I was fascinated by it. It was so simple and uncomplicated. I didn't need to plan exotic menus, buy special diet foods, or measure and count. Frankly, it was revolutionary to me. It was my first taste of freedom, and I liked it a lot.

Never stop any activity because it is "time to eat." "Time to eat" is when your body gives you a real hunger response. All of us have experienced times when we were involved in something interesting or exciting and have inadvertently missed a meal. It was completely painless—we simply became involved in something interesting and forgot to eat.

This concept took me back to my childhood, and I remembered how simple it had all been. I was not heavy as a child. I never gave my weight a thought, yet my weight was always just right. I did remember getting involved in different types of play activities and not even thinking about food until I became very hungry. Then I would eat with a lot of enthusiasm. It was simple; it worked. There was a balance that was so effective that I didn't have to think of it at all.

I began to plan my day without special thought about what I was going to eat. I began to think more about what I was going to do. I found myself able to go for many hours without eating or thinking of food.

Jesus had this effect on people. They often followed to hear Him teach with no thought about what they would eat. In Matthew 14, we are told how the people followed Him from the cities into the desert. He taught and healed their sick all day long. Before they knew it, it was evening, and they were out in the desert with nothing to eat! Over five thousand men, women, and children who did not think about food all day long!

Deal with the Spiritual, Then the Physical

Jesus was moved with compassion, multiplied the five loaves and two fish, and fed over 5,000 people. They all ate until they were *"filled"* (Matthew 14:20). Notice the order of these events. *First,* He dealt with the spiritual—He taught and healed. *Then* and only then did He even think about food.

In Matthew 15, we see Jesus departing to a mountain by the Sea of Galilee. Great multitudes followed Him there as He sat down to teach and heal. We are told that they were filled with wonder *"when they saw the mute speaking, the maimed made whole, the lame walking, and the blind seeing; and they glorified the God of Israel"* (v. 31).

You can imagine their excitement. Perhaps a brother, friend, or neighbor who was deaf was able to hear; a blind person was able to see!

In fact, they were so involved with what God was doing that three days went by! Sometimes we wonder when our pastor talks for one hour! I have a feeling that just about the time someone started to think about food, God worked another mighty miracle. And everyone began glorifying God again and forgot about eating.

Our Lord's Real Concern

After three days, when Jesus finished healing and teaching, He became concerned about the multitudes. *"They have now continued with Me three days and have nothing to eat. And I do not want to send them away hungry, lest they faint on the way"* (Matthew 15:32). You can understand His concern since they still had a long walk back to the coasts of Tyre and Sidon. I love it that Jesus never forgets we live in a human body. He showed us often that He cares about our physical needs. Yet He did not stop ministering just because it was "time to eat."

Two Meals

As I began to eat only from *real hunger,* I soon found that I rarely wanted to eat lunch. I began to plan activities to use the time that I formerly spent planning and eating lunch. I ate breakfast, then dinner. I found that by eating only two meals a day, I could eat whatever I wanted for breakfast and dinner, yet the pounds came off.

Rather than count calories, carbohydrates, or fats, I ate whatever I desired. *But only if I was truly hungry.* I stopped eating when I felt full. I stopped using "diet" products. For the first time I began to eat more satisfying, regular foods. My focus began to change from, "What am I going to *eat* today?" to "What am I going to *do* today?" I began to seek God's purpose for each day and was thrilled to discover He had purpose and meaning for every day.

I began to lose that bloated feeling, "like I needed to drink a bottle of Drano," as one woman so aptly put it. I found I had more energy and more time. I was much more productive and more mentally alert. *That awful, dragging tiredness began to leave.*

Alert on an Empty Stomach

After eating this way for many years, it was interesting for me to read how many ministers and evangelists do not eat before they teach. They say they recall the Word better and are more alert mentally when their stomachs are empty. There are times now, when we have out-of-town company, when I must go back into the three-meals-a-day pattern. Frankly, I always can't wait to get back to two meals a day.

Digesting food is very "labor intensive" for your body. Any athlete knows that your physical endurance is diminished for several hours after a meal. That is because your body is diverted into the task of digesting that food. It has to produce a lot of chemicals, increase blood flow to the digestive area, and store the nutrients. It takes time, it takes energy, and it takes blood flow.

I am astounded by the extent to which we have built our lives around food and eating! Our priorities need to be more like John the Baptist's, who was happy eating locusts and wild honey. There was nothing sacred about eating locusts and wild honey; John ate to live—he didn't live to eat.

I also found that, when eating from *real hunger,* I tended to desire more healthful foods. A person who is having a real hunger response will not desire candy bars or cookies. He will want meat, vegetables, milk, and bread. I eat sweets when I want them; I have dessert when I want it; but I have found my desire for them has diminished. Chocolate doesn't even look good to me most of the time, but if I want some, I eat some. *I just don't eat it to my condemnation anymore.* Praise God!

Hunger Hurts—but Not for Long!

Getting reacquainted with hunger is a learning process. Hunger doesn't last for hours at a time. It comes, makes itself known, and after about fifteen to thirty minutes, it recedes for a long period. That is a good thing to know because there will be times in your healing, when you are gradually extending your times without eating, when you will experience hunger.

Hunger hurts. It is uncomfortable and attention getting. Babies cry when they are hungry because it causes them pain.

If hunger lasted, it would be very difficult to endure for any length of time, *but it doesn't last.* It goes away rather quickly. It is very helpful to get to know how hunger works. If you never "stay it out," you will never understand its characteristics.

I'm telling you ahead of time that it goes away within about half an hour. When it is gone, you feel good again. In fact, you will probably feel *better and more alert* for the next few hours.

It is such a fascinatingly adaptable and perfect response. When a person does feel called by God to fast for several days, he does not wrestle with hunger the entire time. God made it so that when food is not available, there is not a constant, painful urge to eat.

When a person's body is battling an invasion by disease, his hunger response gives place to the more important battle going on. The body needs to focus on producing what is needed to overcome the sickness. People who are ill will say, "I have lost my appetite." What they are expressing is the submission of the hunger response to the more urgent business of the body. When they begin to get better, the hunger comes back. In fact, it is always a good sign when the appetite comes back. It was never really gone; it was just submitting.

You may have periods during your weight loss when you just don't feel hungry. That is because your body is normalizing your weight. You have a more than ample supply of what the body needs, so the hunger recesses temporarily. Your body is using up the stored fat.

Really Enjoying Your Food

When a person begins to eat from hunger instead of the other reasons mentioned, his appetite begins to change. I often prefer a cucumber over anything else. But if I want a chocolate chip cookie, I don't hesitate to eat one. Food is not the culprit—overeating is. *No foods are restricted.* You see, God's plan is freedom. I control my eating; it doesn't control me anymore. I enjoy food much more than I ever did. When you have not eaten since breakfast, dinner looks delicious! I thank God for my food with a sincere heart. I really appreciate it.

The universal reaction as people begin to eat only from *real hunger* is that they experience a new enjoyment of their food. They marvel at the amount of food they were eating when they were not even hungry!

How Did God Feed?

I don't know exactly where today's three-meal-a-day, clean-up-your-plate eating philosophy originated, but it is *not* the pattern that God Himself used when He supernaturally fed men. When we look for spiritual examples of God supernaturally feeding His people, we find a consistent pattern.

In Exodus 16:12, God supernaturally provided food for the Israelites. They were given two meals a day: *"At twilight you shall eat meat, and in the morning you shall be filled with bread."* In fact, their food was provided in such a way that it could be eaten only twice a day even if they wanted to eat three times a day.

We are told that after the morning meal, *"when the sun became hot, it melted"* (v. 21). In the evening they were specifically told to *"let no one leave any of it till morning"* (v. 19). A few of the Israelites, probably the gluttons, decided to try to save a little. They found it had bred worms and begun to stink. That would spoil your appetite for a bedtime snack!

In 1 Kings 17:4–6, we again see an example of God's supernatural feeding. This time He fed His mighty prophet Elijah. Again He gave food twice a day. *"The ravens brought him bread and meat in the morning, and bread and meat in the evening"* (1 Kings 17:6). This time there was neither melting nor breeding of worms, but I am sure Elijah already had his priorities straight as far as eating was concerned. He was eating to live, not living to eat.

When God established the order of the sacrificial offerings in Exodus 29, although He did not supernaturally provide the food, He did set the rules. Again we see His consistent pattern of morning and evening meals. Aaron and his sons were to take their food from certain parts of the sacrificial offering. Bread was to be provided in a basket by the door of the tabernacle of the congregation. *"Then Aaron and his sons shall eat the flesh of the ram, and the bread that is in the basket, by the door of the tabernacle of meeting"* (Exodus 29:32). The sacrifices were offered twice a day. *"One lamb you shall offer in the morning, and the other lamb you shall offer at twilight"* (v. 39).

God's Practicality

There is nothing holy about eating two meals a day or sinful about eating three meals a day. My healing did not come from eating two meals a day; rather, as God healed me, I found myself eating only two meals on most days. Three meals a day would be very uncomfortable for me and feel very unnatural. I often hear people who have been healed of bondage to food say, "I would never go back to eating three meals a day!" I simply believe it is a very practical, good way to eat; and it is the way the Bible says God fed His servants when He was providing the food.

It is readily apparent why this plan would allow a person to eat with more freedom. When you consider the number of calories per day a person may eat to maintain a certain weight, it makes sense. For example, I am 5'9" and weigh 137 pounds. I will be able to eat about 2000 calories a day for the rest of my life. This amount will drop slightly around the age of fifty-five, but basically it will remain the same.

God is not going to change this basic amount of calories because there is nothing wrong with this amount. I am going to need this basic amount of calories for the rest of my natural life. If that 2000 calories is divided three ways, I can eat just over 660 calories per meal.

Typical Meal

For example, a breakfast of cereal with milk and a little sugar has 210 calories. Add orange juice, and you add another 80–100 calories. For lunch, a chef salad (the dieter's favorite) with dressing is about 1000 calories. Add a few crackers—another 50 calories. And because you were so good and ate a salad, you have dessert—another 250 calories, leaving about 400 calories for the evening meal. That means you can eat a delicious meal of thin soup, dry toast, skim milk, and maybe an apple. That's not my idea of a lifetime eating pattern!

With that very same number of calories divided into two meals, there are plenty of calories for you to eat a solid breakfast and still have 1500 calories left over for dinner. This means that going out to dinner will not throw you off, having dessert with your meal will not throw you off, and eating ice cream with the kids will not throw you off. You have real freedom with your eating—freedom to enjoy your food and do as Christ told His disciples: *"Eat such things as are set before you"* (Luke 10:8).

The most important advantage, of course, is that you are no longer counting calories or worrying about which foods are fattening. *You are able to keep your mind off food. Food takes its proper place in your life again.* You begin to eat only when you are hungry and can enjoy the food you eat.

Full Response

When I begin to talk about our equally important full response, people often ask me, "How much can I eat?" You can eat until you are filled. When God fed the Israelites, He said, *"You shall be filled with bread"* (Exodus 16:12). When Jesus multiplied the loaves and fishes, the people *"all ate and were filled"* (Matthew 15:37). Again, in John 6, *"And likewise of the fish, as much as they wanted. So when they were filled, He said to His disciples, 'Gather up the fragments that remain, so that nothing is lost'"* (vv. 11–12).

We should also note that in each case where Jesus multiplied the food, there were *leftovers:* seven basketfuls one time, and twelve basketfuls the other. Eat until you are full, *but no more.* Forget about cleaning up your plate. "Hungry" and "full" are your *God-given* responses. "Clean up your plate" is a *mom-given* response.

People often use the quote "Waste not, want not" with regard to food left on a plate as though it were scriptural. The only problem is that this quote is not from Scripture—it is from Ben Franklin!

Your Individual Response

When Jesus fed the multitudes, in each case He *took up* the fragments so that no food would be wasted. He did not have the people *eat* the fragments so that none would be wasted. In a restaurant, sometimes we are served more food than we can or should eat. Does that mean we should eat it? No! Eat until you are full, but no more.

You will be astonished when you realize how much food you eat only because somebody else put it on your plate. God gave you your hungry and full responses, not the chef at the restaurant or the friend who loaded your plate with food at a dinner party.

Dr. Gabe Mirkin, of the nationally syndicated radio program, put it this way, "When you eat beyond full, all you get is fat!"

Only What Is Sufficient

Sometimes I buy an ice cream cone, and even the smallest can be too much. Other times it is not. If it is too much for me, do I still eat it? No—I eat until I am filled, and no more.

Proverbs 25:16 tells us, *"Have you found honey? Eat only as much as you need."* Again, God gave you your full response, not the ice cream or candy bar makers. Your full response will not remain the same all the time. Just as our caloric needs change, so our full response will change from day to day. Just eat *"as much as you need,"* and don't eat beyond your God-given full response.

Another popular theory used to justify eating beyond our full response is, "Think of the hungry children in India." We should care about the hungry people of the world. Jesus cared when people were hungry. However, the extra food on our plates is not sent to feed the hungry. Our prayers of intercession and God's Word going forth will save the hungry children in India. *The fact that we do or do not clean our plates has absolutely zero effect on the hungry children in India!*

Filled versus Stuffed

If you move into a two-meal-a-day eating pattern, as I did, your appetite will become smaller. You will gradually require less food, although you still will be eating until you are filled. Filled does not mean *stuffed,* but filled does mean you have satisfied your stomach's hunger response.

Whether you eat two meals a day or not, allowing your stomach to become empty is a very important part of your healing. Your natural responses come back in this way. It happens during periods of fasting, when you eat two meals instead of three, or when you get involved in something so interesting or rewarding that you forget to eat.

Healing and freedom do not come from rigid, legalistic rules of eating. Healing and freedom come by bringing God into our relationship with food. In that relationship, we receive help, wisdom, strength, and a supernatural flow of grace that changes our lives, heals our addictions, and ministers to our brokenness.

God will begin to normalize your eating. You will begin to experience and be aware of being full. That is the time to stop eating. It helps to eat a little slower so that your body has time to make the adjustments it was designed to do. In the beginning, eating until you are filled may still require quite a bit of eating. But stop eating when you are filled. The amount will lessen if you are faithful in your daily fasting. You are retraining your body to listen for your God-given hungry and full responses.

It is important to understand that these two responses, hungry and full, operate *in conjunction with one another,* not independent of one another. In other words, in order for your full response to function, you must be hungry when you begin eating. When a person begins to eat without being hungry, he begins to lose his sense of full.

When this happens, there is no full response to shut off the desire for food, and a person continues to eat without reaching a point where he no longer desires food. He continues eating until his stomach is literally stuffed. *This is not a full response.* A full response comes when your body has consumed enough calories to meet its needs.

Response and Desire for Food

When your full response is working properly, you will reach a point where you feel you can't eat another bite. You lose interest in the food, and nothing set before you seems tempting. In fact, the thought of having to eat more food at this time should be somewhat sickening to you. Your response functions as God intended it to; it shuts off your desire for food in a very effective way.

I have watched as people begin to make a decision to stop eating when they are full. In a very short period of time, they are amazed at how much less food they are eating. They are not dieting, not considering what they eat, not feeling guilty or condemned, not denying themselves foods they enjoy, and yet they are losing weight. God really did design us in a way that works beautifully.

In America, where food is so plentiful and servings very large, a full response usually comes before you have eaten everything on your plate. *If you are having seconds on a consistent basis, your full response is not in operation!* A full response probably comes before you have eaten everything on your plate. A stuffed response comes after you have eaten everything on the table!

The Bible calls the latter type of response *"well filled"* as opposed to simply being filled. In Psalm 78:29–31, we see that this type of eating is where gluttony begins.

> *So they ate and were well filled, for He gave them their own desire. They were not deprived of their craving; but while their food was still in their mouths, the wrath of God came against them, and slew the stoutest ["fattest," KJV] of them.*

Taking Up Your Fragments

If you have trouble with continuing to eat even after you are really satisfied, take your plate and run water over it. Make a spiritual intervention by changing something in your physical circumstances for a spiritual purpose. Get the other food off the table as soon as possible. Don't just sit and nibble. Remember that they *took up* the fragments that were left; they did not *eat up* the fragments. (See John 6:12–13.) Take away the food as an act of choosing God in your eating and offer it as seed.

The same principle can be used in a restaurant. If you continue to eat french fries, even when you know you have eaten enough, take your water glass and pour a little water on them. This will kill your appetite for them. The waitress may think you are a little strange, but what do you care if it helps you not to overeat!

Offer it to God. "Father, I choose not to overeat, and I pour this water over these french fries as a way of choosing You in my eating. I offer it to You as seed to the Spirit rather than the flesh."

Although we are born with hungry and full responses and do not have to learn them as children, when we have lost them as adults, *we must relearn them*. We must learn what it feels like to have our stomachs empty—to experience real hunger. Often, after years of dieting, we feel that it is always all right to eat some types of food, such as celery or carrot sticks.

Yet this type of eating, while not high in calories, does not allow you to recognize your hungry and full responses. It does not deal with the gluttony. You are still turning to food, but it is low calorie food instead of high calorie food. It may lead to some control, but never freedom.

Real Hunger Is Easily Satisfied

After having overeaten for many years, most people are amazed at how little food they actually need to eat. Once when I was teaching these principles at my church, a man came to class late and heard only the last thirty minutes of this teaching on hungry and full. He went home, however, and applied what he heard. By the next week he had lost ten pounds by doing nothing but eating only when he was hungry!

People are often astounded to learn they have lost weight by making such a simple change in their lives: don't eat if you aren't hungry. I remember one woman in a group setting who gave excuses all the way to being weighed on the scale. She said that all she did was not eat when she wasn't hungry, and that she probably hadn't lost any weight. Her face certainly came alive when she saw she had lost three pounds that week and didn't even know it!

When people have struggled so much with their weight, drawing on all their willpower and constraining themselves to the very limit of their endurance to take off weight, they are utterly unprepared for the "easy yoke" when Jesus is in it with them. I frequently receive calls from people expressing concern because it is too easy. They actually want to know what is wrong!

Drastic Drop in Appetite

People also become concerned when they have a drastic decrease in appetite. This excerpt from a letter I recently received is an example of how people frequently respond to such a result. "I felt I wasn't getting enough to eat! I could eat only half a banana and half a sandwich, and that was a challenge." Another lady, who had over sixty pounds to lose, said she was worried because she could eat only about half of what was on her plate.

A person who is sixty pounds overweight has 210,000—or *almost a quarter of a million*—stored calories (in the form of fat). *Expect a drastic decrease in your appetite* as you begin to eat based on your God-given hungry and full responses. Count on it—watch for it—rejoice in it!

The following chart will help you understand why your appetite will decrease significantly. It also helps illustrate why too much weight is a strain on the body and why it saps vital energy.

Stored Calories per Pound of Overweight by Diane Hampton

Pounds of Overweight	Stored Calories of Fat	Days of Stored Calories	Months of Stored Calories
5	17,500	8.75	
10	35,000	17.5	
15	52,500	26.25	
20	70,000	35.00	1.1
25	87,500	43.75	1.45
30	105,000	52.5	1.72
35	122,500	61.25	2.00
40	140,000	70.00	2.30
45	157,500	78.75	2.58
50	175,000	87.50	2.87
55	192,500	96.25	3.15
60	210,000	105.00	3.44
65	227,500	113.75	3.73
70	245,000	122.50	4.02
75	262,500	131.25	4.30
80	280,000	140.00	4.59
85	297,500	148.75	4.88
90	315,000	157.50	5.16

95	332,500	166.25	5.45
100	350,000	175.00	5.73
105	367,500	183.75	6.02
110	385,000	192.50	6.31

These computations are based on caloric needs of approximately 2000 calories a day and 3500 calories per one pound of excess weight.

While our bodies store fat, *they cannot store many needed vitamins.* Just because you have a month's worth of stored fat does not mean you have a month's worth of stored vitamins and minerals. However, this chart helps us understand the decrease in appetite and feel more comfortable with it.

The "Easy Yoke"

A few years ago, my husband and I went on a cruise. Anyone who has been on a cruise knows the lavish meals they serve. Every meal was a feast! Toward the end of the cruise, some of the passengers were waddling on the decks, stuffed to the gills, yet dreading the inevitable diets they anticipated on their return home. I ate anything I wanted throughout the entire cruise and thoroughly enjoyed the food, but I didn't gain a pound.

Before I went in for a meal, I considered, "Am I really hungry?" If the answer was "No," I did not even go into the dining room. This almost always occured at the noon meal. Don and I would walk the decks, shop, or do something else.

When evening came, we were ready to eat! I'll bet our food tasted better than anyone else's because we allowed ourselves to become hungry before we ate. It is not unusual for people to write me that they had been on vacation and yet still lost weight. They lost this weight even though they ate every meal at a restaurant!

One woman reported that she had lost three pounds over her vacation. And she never ate any special foods or diet menus. *Freedom.* Another woman, over forty years of age, reported that for the first time in her life, she did not gain weight over the Thanksgiving holiday. Yet she ate everything to her satisfaction and without that awful guilt.

Compensating for a Large Meal

Eating only when you are hungry, after having eaten a large meal the previous evening, can mean not eating until the evening meal the next day. You will not become hungry until your body needs fuel again, and that will be longer than normal when you have eaten a large amount. In other words, if you have eaten more than your daily caloric needs in one meal, don't eat with your usual pattern the next day. Allow your body to use up the extra calories by waiting until you are hungry.

Some Common Changes

Once, in a group, I asked the men and women to write down some of the changes that had come about in their lives as they had begun to make alterations in their eating habits that were bringing healing in their lives.

Over and over they mentioned they had more fellowship with God. They found that they easily adjusted to fewer meals; they were more active, more productive, had a new enjoyment for life, were more obedient in other areas, watched less TV, and found it much easier to fast when they were called to fast for other reasons.

They also mentioned how their faith had grown to believe God for other things as they saw victory in their weight. The direction and focus of their lives changed from food to fellowship. They began to become much more fruitful in their lives.

In Mark 4, Jesus taught the parable of parables. By this I mean that He said, *"Do you not understand this parable? How then will you understand all the parables?"* (v. 13). He seemed to give special emphasis to one parable and to be telling us that it is foundational to understanding basic things about God's kingdom.

In verses 16–17, He said that for the seed to grow, there must be a root system. *"Who, when they hear the word, immediately receive it with gladness; and they have no root in themselves, and so endure only for a time."* He is saying that we must have a root system in ourselves. Roots stabilize a plant and reach down into the soil to bring nutrients and moisture. He is speaking of our relationship with God. If we don't have that relationship, the word sown is falling on stony ground.

Then in Mark 4:19, He spoke of the seed sown among thorns. *"The cares of this world, the deceitfulness of riches, and the desires for other things entering in choke the word, and it becomes unfruitful."* When we lust after food, the word sown can be choked in our lives.

In this same chapter of Mark, Jesus said,

> *To what shall we liken the kingdom of God? Or with what parable shall we picture it? It is like a mustard seed which, when it is sown on the ground, is smaller than all the seeds on earth;* ***but when it is sown****, it grows up and becomes greater than all herbs.* (vv. 30–32, emphasis added)

Don't underestimate the power of small seeds of faith, small spiritual interventions in your eating where you "sow" spiritual seed. Jesus said, *"When it is sown on the ground, is smaller than all the seeds on earth; but* ***when it is sown, it grows****."* These seemingly small changes will bring an incredible harvest of healing.

Small seeds bring great victories, and God is glorified.

Right now, you may be experiencing something deep inside you that you know is God-breathed. It is a seed of hope. "Maybe I can be free. Maybe it is possible." You can. For the past twenty years, I have received letters from all over the world. People tell me that their lives have been changed. "For the first time, I am free." "This book changed my life!" A woman in South Africa was so excited about her newfound freedom that she started a clinic to help others learn from her new success.

Chapter 5

Resisting Temptation

Scripture tells us, *"Therefore submit to God"* (James 4:7). You are learning a lot of ways to submit your eating to God. When you offer these spiritual seeds to God, you are submitting yourself and your eating to Him. It is a good thing to make a habit of speaking certain things out loud. For one thing, when you speak something out loud, you have more than doubled its effectiveness in your life because you have now heard it spoken, as well as read it. For this reason, it can be very helpful and faith-building to tell God you are submitting your eating to Him this day. "Father, I choose You in my eating today. I choose Your will for my life. I will sow seed to the Spirit this day and not to the flesh."

The second part of this Scripture says, *"Resist the devil and he will flee from you."* To resist means to "strive against or oppose, to make a stand or effort in opposition." It does not necessarily mean to stand in a nose-to-nose confrontation. If you sit and think about a piece of blueberry pie to see how long you can hold out, you're not going to make it very long.

A saying that has been around for a long time with regard to parenting advises, "Choose your battles!" It's a good thing to remember as you seek to bring your eating into the freedom that God wants you to have. There is a time and place to choose your battles.

Eating and Non-Eating Activities

As we draw near to God, He draws near to us (James 4:8). One of the many ways that God manifests Himself is with gifts of wisdom or knowledge. This knowledge is not acquired by study or learned. It is given. It is just deposited into your spirit by His Spirit. These gifts of knowledge really make a difference in our circumstances. The expression, "It just came to me out of the blue!" is the way we often feel when the Holy Spirit drops an answer into our spirits.

His answers or gifts of knowledge are usually quite succinct and are always powerful when implemented in our lives. I recall a pastor telling me once of something God had showed him that was truly powerful. I have never forgotten it because it was so filled with wisdom. He said, "God showed me this one time. Every message is a love message. It says, 'I love you' or it says, 'Do you love me?'" This wisdom was customized for him. It was especially important to this pastor because he is an engineer by education and by mind-set. This makes him especially weak in the area of human relationships, so God gave him a gift of knowledge to help him minister. When he incorporates this wisdom into his ministry, he becomes much more effective.

God gave me simple, powerful, customized truths that were foundational to my healing and continued freedom. God showed me that there were certain times and activities, certain things that I did, when I consistently tended to overeat.

Understanding this allowed me to set some boundaries for my freedom. For example, I tended to overeat when I was alone. I tended to overeat after a certain time in the evening, like after 9:00 PM. I tended to overeat when I was tired. These were things I had control over, but until God allowed me to see them, I wasn't even aware of them. I could choose to go to bed earlier. I could choose not to be alone in the house. It was a matter of choosing my battles, and I could win these. Winnable skirmishes!

Conversely, there were certain times and activities when I consistently tended to forget about eating. For example, I could be talking to a friend and not even think about eating. I could be involved in a fun sewing project and not even think about food.

Take a moment and begin to consider your life. When do you overeat? Is there a certain time of day when you are more vulnerable? Where do you overeat? Is there a certain location in your house where you are more vulnerable? Who is with you when you overeat? What do you have control over in your situation?

It would be worthwhile for you to take a sheet of paper and make a list called, "Activities When I Consistently Tend to Overeat." Allow this list to be deeply incorporated into your spirit. Here are just three of many verses that reinforce the importance of setting these boundaries.

> *Do not enter the path of the wicked, and do not walk in the way of evil* [a situation that usually leads to overeating]. *Avoid it, do not travel on it; turn away from it and pass on.* (Proverbs 4:14–15)

> *Ponder the path of your feet, and let all your ways be established.* (Proverbs 4:26)

> *The highway of the upright is to depart from evil; he who keeps his way preserves his soul.*
> (Proverbs 16:17)

All these Scriptures speak about guarding and regarding your path. Think about where you are going, what you are doing. Ponder the path of your feet. Your feet may be taking you to the refrigerator when you know you are bored, not hungry.

Your feet may be walking your body over to the sofa to sit down and turn on the TV when you know it will lead to eating. Establish your path by telling your feet to take you someplace else! They will do what you tell them to when you consciously enter into the decision.

For many, many years I drove our two daughters in a car pool with a couple of other families. It was a habit because I repeated it for so many years. I was like a trail horse; I could follow the "car pool trail" without even thinking about it. Our bodies and minds adjust to these habitual things so that we don't have to reinvent the wheel, so to speak, each time we do a repeated activity.

One summer, the girls changed schools, and I no longer had to drive in the car pool. I could not count the number of times that I caught myself getting in the car and mechanically beginning to drive the route I had taken for the car pool! I would realize that I was heading in the direction of the old familiar stops rather than where I should have been heading! It was a habit that had been formed over many years, and I sometimes unconsciously fell back into it.

You have eating habits like this. You have little pathways that have been ingrained into your daily routine. It is going to take a conscious effort to change these habits.

That is why it is valuable to do something like actually sitting down and writing out these pathways that lead to overeating. A teacher may have students write something over and over. That won't necessarily change their behavior, *but it will sure make them think more about their decisions.*

I have recently been meeting with a beautiful young Christian woman. She is a new believer and is like a sponge in her hunger for God and His Word. We have been meeting to help her with her weight.

The first time we met, I told her that we were not going to be talking about food. She seemed a little surprised. Instead I gave her some things that Jesus said about being free and about nothing being impossible with God. I had her write them down and read them during the week.

The second week, we again looked up Scriptures that gave testimony to how God works in our lives. We read about seeds and sowing and reaping. We read about how the Holy Spirit brings truth, and so on. We never talked about food.

The third week, we talked about this issue of "pondering" (thinking about) the path of our feet. She had a real breakthrough week. She said, "I put a reminder on my refrigerator to think about where my feet were going. When I saw it, I would stop and think about what I was doing. I would decide to do something else. It was so easy. I couldn't believe it could be this easy to lose weight." She lost three pounds that week.

Think about how hard it is to diet and restrict what you eat. Think about all the special foods you need to buy and the preparations you must make. Think about how you couldn't wait to get off the diet!

Compare that to this simple change in the way you approach your decisions. The weight loss is the same. Very few diets would produce a consistent weight loss of two to three pounds a week, yet here she was, losing weight, but not restricting what she ate.

God is smart. He is really, really smart, and He knows how to bring you into freedom.

It is equally important to think about times and activities when you tend not to overeat. What are you doing when you aren't tempted to overeat? Where are you? Who are you with? What time of day is it?

The value of making this list is, again, to help renew your mind with regard to eating. By thinking about it and writing it down, you are beginning to change your thought processes about food.

It prepares you for those times of temptation. If you tend to overeat when you are tired, for example, that is probably not a good time to have to think up an alternative plan of action.

When you are learning to change your thought processes, this is not a time when you have to impress God with your spirituality. It is the motivation behind your action that God will be interested in. You could be doing something that looks insignificant to others, but is very significant to God. If you are tired and headed straight for the kitchen, choosing to take a bubble bath instead can have a great impact on your healing. This is because this choice is really a spiritual intervention in your life where you do something natural for a "supernatural" reason. You changed the path of your feet so that you would not be led into temptation.

This list should include some activities that don't take a lot of time or money. Some of the activities should include projects that are creative and interesting, such as making a quilt or doing a flower arrangement. For the list to be valuable, however, it needs to include activities that are simple to implement—activities that don't require any kind of shopping list.

The following are practical examples of the kinds of things that could be on your list. (Their common denominator is that they all tend to lead away from overeating.)

1. Playing the piano or other musical instrument
2. Going for a walk outside
3. Listening to a teaching tape
4. Cleaning out a closet or drawer
5. Making a list of future projects
6. Having coffee with a friend
7. Writing letters or thank-you notes
8. Doing laundry and ironing
9. Manicuring and painting your fingernails
10. Giving yourself a facial (Oatmeal and water make a great one!)
11. Sweeping the garage
12. Driving to the park
13. Sketching or painting
14. Reading a magazine
15. Working a puzzle

By taking the time to make out this list ahead of time, you can put it on the refrigerator and glance at it when needed. Again, the list should include a wide variety of possibilities. It should have things that can be done alone as well as with other people. It should include activities that are fun as well as functional and activities that may require some expense as well as some that don't require any expense.

One way of sowing to the Spirit and resisting the devil is to consciously choose to move from an "eating activity" to a "non-eating activity." If you have trouble with eating when you are in your house alone, one way of sowing to the Spirit is to choose to get out of your house (go visit a friend in the hospital, take a walk around the block) and offer it to God as seed. "Father, You know that I would like to eat right now, but I choose to get out of the house instead, and I offer this to You as seed."

If you have trouble with snacking too much when you watch TV at night, choose to do handiwork or take a bath instead.

Choosing to Sow Seed

There is nothing holy about taking a walk or doing handiwork. It is when you purposely choose to do these activities instead of eating and offer them to God as a way of choosing Him in your eating that you have sown seed to the Spirit. Proverbs 16:2 tells us, *"All the ways of a man are pure in his own eyes, but the LORD weighs the spirits."* Avoid activities that usually lead to overeating, even if they seem right with your natural eye. God *"weighs the spirits"*; He knows that you know the activities lead to overeating.

Get your focus off what you are eating or not eating. Focus on which activities lead to eating and which activities do not. As God begins to reveal this to you, use your power of choice wisely. The Bible clearly teaches that the choices we make affect our freedom.

Understanding and Wisdom from God

One of the ways I was able to control overeating was to stop staying up late at night. I liked to watch the late movie. In fact, I learned that any time I stayed up late, I was much more likely to overeat the next day. Once I understood this, I began to *"ponder the path of* [my] *feet"* (Proverbs 4:26) and establish my way. I did this by going to bed earlier instead of watching the late movie. Now, there is nothing wrong with staying up late at night, but the *"LORD weighs the spirits"* (Proverbs 16:2), and for me, keeping late hours led to overeating.

With my healing, I received wisdom from God with regard to my eating. My healing has continued over twenty years because God gave me wisdom.

> *From His mouth come knowledge and understanding* [with regard to eating]*; He stores up sound wisdom for the upright; He is a shield to those who walk uprightly; He guards the paths of justice, and preserves the way of His saints. Then you will understand righteousness* [He not only healed me, but He also showed me how He intended me to eat, what type of eating leads to gluttony, and what type does not]....*When wisdom enters your heart, and knowledge is pleasant to your soul, discretion will preserve you; understanding will keep you.* (Proverbs 2:6–11)

What Is Discretion?

Discretion means the freedom or authority to make decisions and choices. God's Word says that this discretion will preserve you. When you are trapped in a food addiction—or any compulsive behavior—your choices are hidden from you. God returns your freedom of choice, but He leaves the final choice with you. Your discretion will keep, or preserve, you in freedom. I know that I will never have a problem with eating again for the rest of my life because I make choices every day according to the wisdom God gave me regarding food. How much better to have understanding and weight loss rather than just weight loss.

Keeping Your House Clean

Jesus warned us,

> *When an unclean spirit goes out of a man* [such as the spirit of overeating], *he goes through dry places, seeking rest, and finds none. Then he says, "I will return to my house from which I came* [your heart and mind]." *And when he comes, he finds it empty* [still sitting there, watching TV, thinking about food], *swept, and put in order* [ripe for a binge]. *Then he goes and takes with him seven other spirits more wicked than himself* [Mr. Binge, Mr. Condemnation, Mr. Depression, and so on], *and they enter and dwell there; and the last state of that man is worse than the first.* (Matthew 12:43–45)

Don't let Satan come back to find your house empty! Let him find you full of the Word and moving out in faith to another activity. Resist the devil. If you resist, he must flee from you.

Changing from eating to non-eating activities is not just a good thing to do, but *it is also a vital part of your healing.* Jesus warns us in this parable from Matthew 12 that if we leave our house empty, if we don't fill that part of our life with something meaningful, then we are open prey for the same wicked spirits to return, stronger than before.

How to Change Your Ways

If you have trouble because you eat after dinner, night after night, *repent!* To repent means to "think differently." Change the way you think about your time after dinner. Start taking walks, play a family game, or start a hobby that keeps your hands busy. Replace the old, negative pattern in your life with something positive. Plan other activities during the time you used to have a problem with eating.

For example, I always try to schedule all appointments around the noon hour. This is an old habit I picked up during the time of my healing (sow an action; reap a habit). I learned that if I had an activity planned for the time I had trouble with eating, I would fast much more easily. I learned to "keep my way" in order to preserve my soul.

Choosing the Right Activity

Make your activity something you can look forward to. As much as possible, make it involve other people. Be creative in your ideas. I found that planning more activities outside in the fresh air helped.

Sometimes we must fill our empty house with the Word of God. David said of God, *"You are my hiding place; You shall preserve me from trouble; You shall surround me with songs of deliverance....Whenever I am afraid, I will trust in You"* (Psalms 32:7; 56:3). God's Word is our "song of deliverance." Our souls can hide in it when we are afraid.

When I was worried, instead of turning to food, as I had before, I listened to a Christian teaching tape or worship music, or I read the Bible or books about the Bible. *"Trust in the LORD with all your heart, and lean not on your own understanding"* (Proverbs 3:5). God's Word ministered to my spirit, and I was able to stop worrying. When I felt depression coming, instead of eating, I read, *"For God has not given us a spirit of fear, but of power and of love and of a sound mind"* (2 Timothy 1:7).

Instead of fighting with a knife and fork, I began to do battle with the sword of the Word. It ministered to my spirit, and I was able to resist depression.

When I was angry at others or myself, instead of eating I would read, *"Renew a right spirit within me"* (Psalm 51:10 KJV), and *"If you do not forgive men their trespasses, neither will your Father forgive your trespasses"* (Matthew 6:15). Formerly, I always said in my heart, "God knows why I am angry. He knows what they did to me. I don't get mad without a good reason." When I saw from God's Word that Scripture didn't mention whether or not I had a good reason, I became serious about forgiving.

I found that as I began to forgive others, I was able to forgive myself. God's Word is health, purity, truth, and righteousness.

A Just Man Falls Seven Times

What if you begin the day, commit your eating to God, and all goes well until about 10:00 AM? Then you begin to eat. My healing was not overnight. It took a period of months, and sometimes I fell back into binges during those months.

What do you do if you fall? And you can expect that you will. Perfection is God's exclusive attribute. When you do disappoint yourself, remember that God doesn't work through perfection, He works through repentance. You can expect that condemning, discouraging thoughts will come to you. Satan is called the *"accuser of our brethren"* (Revelation 12:10). He literally brings discouraging, self-hating thoughts to try to separate you from God and His healing power. He tries to convince you that God has given up on you with thoughts like, "You'll never be free. Here you go again, same old eating, same old failure. You have blown it now. You'll never get back to where you were. God's not going to help you after this binge!"

God, on the other hand, understands that progress may be three steps forward and two steps back in the very beginning. He reveals in His Word that He doesn't give up on us. I love what Proverb 24:16 says: *"For a righteous man may fall seven times and rise again."* That tells me that

God often cuts us a lot more slack than we cut ourselves! A baby falls over and over when he is learning to walk. Sometimes he cries, and at first he looks pretty confused when he falls. Then he learns that it is all right to fall if he gets right back up and tries again. The result is that he learns to walk.

Being perfect before God is not a matter of never falling—*it is a question of what you do about it when you do fall.* A just man rises up again!

Why do you think condemnation is such a favorite tool of the devil? Because he knows if he can get you into condemnation rather than repentance, he can probably keep you from turning to God. Satan likes nothing better than to tell us we have really blown it, and that we had better not go to God after what we've done.

When we have overeaten (or done anything else sinful), we feel the least like going before God. We don't even want to be around other people. But this is the most important time to go to God.

Is It Too Late for a New Beginning?

You have not blown it. You are not on a diet, so you can't blow it! Tell yourself, "I have sown to the flesh, but I will not say that I have blown it and continue to sow to the flesh. I repent, Father, and I resolve right now, *this hour,* to sow to the Spirit. I thank You, Father, that it is never too late for a new beginning. This day may have started in defeat, but it will end in victory!"

Remember the woman who was caught in the act of adultery? People wanted to stone her, but when she was brought before Jesus, He said, *"Neither do I condemn you: go, and sin no more"* (John 8:11). If you will go to God right in the middle of a binge and repent, His answer will be the same. *"Neither do I condemn you,"* and you will be able to *"go and sin no more."*

You see, when that woman repented, she chose Jesus, and power was released into her life to go and sin no more. That same power will be released into your life. You have God's Word on it. He promised, *"But as many as received Him, to them He gave the right* [*"power,"* KJV] *to become children of God"* (John 1:12). Purpose in your heart to commit your eating to God, and redirect the focus of your life away from food.

God Has a Plan for Your Life

On subsequent pages are what we call "Seven Days of Recreating Your Eating Patterns." Each day there is a prayer to commit that day's eating to God. There is a space to write down what you resolve to do that day instead of eating. It is important for your success that you decide each day what you are going to do as seed to the Spirit.

In the past, you have spent much time and planning on what you were going to *eat.* Now spend some time planning what you are going to *do.* Remember that God has a purpose and plan for each life, and binge eating is not on His "to do" list. God gives purpose and dignity to our lives. He allows us to see and serve others in a way that benefits everyone.

When you make your weekly plan, don't forget to include those things that Jesus values. He gives us so many examples in the Bible of ways He wants us to help others. The parable of the Good Samaritan tells us to take time to help hurting people wherever we find them. The message is, "Don't get so busy—even with church work—that you pass them by." It was a priest and Levite who didn't stop to help.

> *Now by chance a certain priest came down that road. And when he saw him, he passed by on the other side. Likewise a Levite, when he arrived at the place, came and looked, and passed by on the other side.* (Luke 10:31–32)

Jesus pointed out the needy, impoverished people of the world and said,

> *I was hungry and you gave Me food; I was thirsty and you gave Me drink; I was a stranger and you took Me in; I was naked and you clothed Me; I was sick and you visited Me; I was in prison and you came to Me.* (Matthew 25:35–36)

In the last ten years, my husband and I have had the opportunity to travel to many of the needy areas of the world. In Zimbabwe, Africa, I literally gave a drink of water "in His name" as we passed out food and tin cups of water to the hungry who gathered at night in the streets of Harare.

In Kosovo, we helped to build shelters as the frigid winter approached. Hundreds of thousands had come back after the fighting to find their homes destroyed and often their husbands, fathers, brothers, and uncles murdered. There is a world out there that many Americans have never dreamed of.

God Bless America

I was deeply touched, however, to find something out about this wonderful country of ours as I traveled to Harare, Zimbabwe. It took thirty-two hours of travel to get there from St. Louis. On the last leg of the flight, from London to Harare, I expected to find many empty seats. Instead, there were none! I kept thinking, "Why would all these people be going to Zimbabwe? It has the highest rate of AIDS in the world, its economy is in shambles with 70 percent unemployment, and its currency is worthless. Why, why, why are all these people on this plane?" During the twelve hour flight, I had an opportunity to talk to a number of the other passengers. What I found out touched me deeply and made me so proud to be an American.

That plane was filled to capacity because of all the Americans who were going to Zimbabwe to give aid to these precious people in His name. They came from Nebraska, Pennsylvania, Oklahoma, Missouri and who knows how many other places. The newspapers and news media didn't report it, but I kept thinking, "God, You see this, don't You?" Inwardly, I was singing,

God bless America, land that I love,
Stand beside her and guide her
Through the night with the light from above.

We have gotten only small glimpses of what Jesus must have seen from His eternal perspective as He spoke those words from Matthew 25 shortly before His death. We don't have to do all our planned activities of service in one week or one month, but rather steadily incorporating them over the course of our lifetimes, so that when we stand before Him, our lives will have given evidence of His love.

Our planned activities can include many other things, as well. We are given the overall job description of "subduing the earth and taking dominion over it." (See Genesis 1:28.) That could mean cleaning out a closet or just going to work at your job as a secretary or accountant. It could include teaching someone something. It could be meeting a new neighbor or doing handiwork.

One of your activities can be your commitment to read confessions each day about your eating. That is nothing more than letting your mouth speak what you believe so that your ears can hear it, and your mind can be renewed by it.

The Rule of Twenty-One

At the end of the week, go back and see how successful you have been in reaching your goals. Give yourself a grade, and then do the same thing the next week. It takes about twenty-one days to establish a new pattern in your life.

I wear something called "mono-vision" contact lenses. That means that I wear two very different corrections in my eyes. One lets me read and the other lets me drive. It works very well for me, but in the beginning I saw double. The doctor told me that it would take about twenty-one days for my brain to become adjusted to the new way of seeing. Actually, it didn't take quite that long, but he was right in telling me that my brain would adjust.

Your brain needs to develop a new way of seeing your life and relationship with food. You may see double in the beginning—the way you used to see and respond to food and the way you are now seeing and responding to food. That double vision will become single vision if you stay in there.

Don't leave these spaces blank. Decide what seeds you are going to sow each day, write them in, then do them. If you begin to fall back into poor eating habits, don't let Satan tell you where you have failed for the day. Start from that hour as though it were a new day.

One of the greatest joys I had during my time of healing was when I began a binge, realized what I was doing, and then made a decision to choose God. I never finished the binge. That was when I knew I was being healed.

Day 1

Begin with a prayer of humble dependence on God's gracious kindness and power to bring healing. Use your own words or these words: "Father, I thank You for making healing possible for me. I invite You into my eating today, and I open the doors of my heart. I don't want to hold back any part of me from Your love. Will You help me today to be sensitive to Your promptings and insight with regard to my eating? Will You help me to see the holy purpose that You have for my life? I believe that these next three weeks will change my life because, with You, God, nothing is impossible. Amen."

Seed to the Spirit:

Instead of eating lunch or dinner (circle one) this day I will ________________________, and I offer this to You, Lord, as seed to the Spirit.

Instead of bedtime eating this day I will ________________________, and I offer this to You, Lord, as seed to the Spirit.

I will offer thanksgiving to You for everything I eat today because Your Word says that my food is sanctified by this thanksgiving. (See 1 Timothy 3:1, 3–4.)

I will read my confessions from Your Word this day and my confessions about my weight.

Day 2

Father, I commit my eating to You today. Fill this day with Your purpose and meaning. I will sow seed to the Spirit today to set a new eating pattern in my life. I receive You this day in my eating, and I receive power to walk as a child of God. Father, I thank You that Your Word is supernatural. Because it is supernatural, I will have supernatural help when I choose You in my eating.

Seed to the Spirit:

Instead of eating lunch or dinner (circle one) this day I will ______________________, and I offer this to You, Lord, as seed to the Spirit.

Instead of bedtime eating this day I will ______________________, and I offer this to You, Lord, as seed to the Spirit.

I will offer thanksgiving to You for everything I eat today because Your Word says my food is sanctified by this thanksgiving.

I will read positive confessions about my eating today, and I will meditate on Your Word when I am lonely, worried, frustrated, angry, or experiencing other negative emotions.

Day 3

Father, I commit my eating to You today. Beginning this day, I will seek a new eating pattern for me that will last for the rest of my life. I will seek a change in my whole attitude about food and my appetite. Your Word says that *"he who sows to the Spirit will of the Spirit reap"* (Galatians 6:8). So I offer You my seed to eat only two meals this day. You promised power to as many as received You. I receive You this day in my eating, and I receive power to walk as a child of God in my eating.

Seed to the Spirit:

Instead of eating lunch or dinner (circle one) this day I will ______________________, and I offer this to You, Lord, as seed to the Spirit.

Instead of bedtime eating this day I will __________________________, and I offer this to You, Lord, as seed to the Spirit.

I will offer thanksgiving to You for everything I eat today because Your Word says my food is sanctified by this thanksgiving.

I will read my confessions from Your Word this day and my confessions about my weight.

Day 4

Father, I commit my eating to You today. Fill this day with Your purpose and meaning. I will sow seed to the Spirit today to set a new eating pattern in my life. I receive You this day in my eating, and I receive power to walk as a child of God in my eating. Father, I thank You that Your Word is supernatural, so that I will have supernatural help when I choose You in my eating.

Seed to the Spirit:

Instead of eating lunch or dinner (circle one) this day I will __________________________, and I offer this to You, Lord, as seed to the Spirit.

Instead of bedtime eating this day I will __________________________, and I offer this to You, Lord, as seed to the Spirit.

I will offer thanksgiving to You for everything I eat today because Your Word says my food is sanctified by this thanksgiving.

I will read my confessions about my eating today, and I will meditate on Your Word when I am lonely, frustrated, worried, angry, or experiencing any other negative emotion.

Day 5

Father, I commit my eating to You today. I choose obedience. Jesus said, *"If you love Me, keep My commandments"* (John 14:15), and I love You, Lord, so I will not eat to my condemnation. I will sow seed to the Spirit so that I may reap of the Spirit.

Seed to the Spirit:

Instead of eating lunch or dinner (circle one) this day I will __________________________, and I offer it to You, Lord, as seed to the Spirit.

Instead of bedtime eating this day I will __________________________, and I offer this to You, Lord, as seed to the Spirit.

I will offer thanksgiving to You for everything I eat today because Your Word says my food is sanctified by this thanksgiving.

I will read positive confessions about my eating today, and I will meditate on Your Word when I am lonely, worried, frustrated, or angry.

Day 6

Father, I commit my eating to You today. You know that this is a weekend, Father, so I ask for special help today. I ask You for special purpose for this day. I will sow seed to the Spirit today and expect to reap from the Spirit. I receive You in my eating today, and I thank You for power to walk as a child of God in my eating this day.

Seed to the Spirit:

Instead of eating lunch or dinner (circle one) I will ________________________, and I offer this to You, Lord, as seed to the Spirit.

Instead of bedtime eating this day I will ________________________, and I offer this to You, Lord, as seed to the Spirit.

I will offer thanksgiving to You for everything I eat today because Your Word says my food is sanctified by this thanksgiving.

I will read my confessions about my eating today from Your Word.

Day 7

The seventh day is God's day of rest. It is a gift to you from your Father in heaven.

Dear God, thank You for all you are doing in my life right now. Thank You for the changes I am beginning to experience in my thoughts and relationship with food and eating. I acknowledge and rejoice that You are changing me for the rest of my life.

What to Expect from Your Seed

When you plant a seed in the ground, it will not come up the next day. In fact, you will not see anything happen for a week to ten days. You have to watch and believe the seed is growing. After a week or ten days, you begin to see a tiny sprout pushing up out of the ground.

It will be the same with your fasting. There will be a time at the beginning when it will seem as if nothing is happening. That is the time you must stand in faith. Do not stop making your daily commitment to God. God's Word says something will happen, *and it will happen.*

After a time, you will begin to see the "sprout" in your life, and you will notice that food is losing its control over you. Chocolate will stop looking so good. Things that were hard to pass up will become easier and easier not to eat. You will begin to be free indeed.

When to Set Fasting Goals

If at any point the fasting becomes too heavy, go back to the hungry and full pattern. If you find yourself setting fasting goals you are not meeting, go back to asking yourself before you eat anything, "Am I really hungry?" Don't set a fasting goal for yourself at this time.

When Jesus is in the yoke with you, fasting will not be a difficult thing. Remember, Jesus said that if we are faithful in that which is least, we will be faithful in much. (See Luke 16:10.) Go back to where you can be faithful and be sensitive to the change in your appetite when it comes. You will begin to experience a supernatural ability to fast. That is the time to get back to fasting.

Chapter 6

Transformed by New Thoughts

Most Christians have heard Mark 11:23 quoted many times.

> *Whoever says to this mountain, "Be removed and be cast into the sea," and does not doubt in his heart, but believes that those things he says will be done, he will have whatever he says.*

It is one of the great truths of God.

But did you know this same truth can work in a negative way? Remember when Jesus walked by the fig tree without fruit, and He cursed it by saying, *"Let no one eat fruit from you ever again"* (v. 14)? I used to wonder why Jesus would curse a poor old fig tree. He was teaching us that faith can work in a negative way, also. The next day when the disciples passed the fig tree, they marveled because it had dried up from the roots, but Jesus said, *"He will have whatever he says."*

Cursing Your Fig Tree

Some people have been cursing their fig trees with regard to their weight for many years. "I just can't seem to lose weight. I came from an overweight family. I guess I will always be fat. I can look at food and gain weight." Yet Proverbs 13:2 says, *"A man shall eat well by the fruit of his mouth."* Proverbs 18:20 says, *"A man's stomach shall be satisfied from the fruit of his mouth."*

Paul's admonition in Romans 12:2 to *"not be conformed to this world, but be transformed by the renewing of your mind"* coincides with the truth that our words are creative. If we renew our minds and uplift our thoughts, our words will also be uplifting.

Some words build us up inside. When I am discouraged, or something seems overwhelming to me, I say, *"I can do all things through Christ who strengthens me"* (Philippians 4:13). That Scripture reaches down inside me and lifts me up. My posture gets a little straighter, and I know I am going to make it. I have done things I would have sworn were impossible by stepping out in faith on this Scripture.

Some words fill up your soul. Proverbs 27:7 tells us, *"A satisfied soul loathes the honeycomb."* If your soul is full, even a honeycomb (today it might be a milk chocolate bar) isn't tempting. This proverb also warns, *"To a hungry soul every bitter thing is sweet."*

If your soul is hungry, if you feel turmoil inside, you will want to eat everything. Even unappetizing things will seem sweet. Therefore, when you feel discouragement emptying your soul, have some food for the soul ready.

Words to Fill Your Soul

Saying, "I can't seem to lose weight" empties your soul. Saying, *"The things which are impossible with men are possible with God"* (Luke 18:27) fills your soul. Instead of saying, "I can't seem to lose weight," say, "I lose weight easily." Instead of saying, "I have been overweight all my life," say, "I am being changed by the power of God." Here are some more positive faith statements about weight that you might use:

> *"I can do all things through Christ who strengthens me"* (Philippians 4:13). I can lose weight and control my eating for the rest of my life through Christ.
>
> My appetite is being totally changed through Jesus my Lord. Jesus *"Himself bore* [my] *sins in His own body…that* [I]*…might live for righteousness"* (1 Peter 2:24) and be dead to every form of bondage.
>
> I receive Jesus in my eating, so I receive *"power to…*[fill in the blank] *of God"* (John 1:12 KJV).
>
> I will soon wear a size ______ dress or suit.
>
> I will weigh _______ pounds because I can lose weight easily now.

You may use any of these positive words or make up a list of your own. Begin to repeat healing Scriptures aloud each day. Apply them to your weight. Jesus said, *"For out of the abundance of the heart the mouth speaks. A good man out of the good treasure of his heart brings forth good things"* (Matthew 12:34–35).

Old Things Are Passed Away

The devil is called the deceiver. He often tries to lead us into spiritual quicksand where we can get stuck. If we don't know the Word of God, we will begin to sink. There is a teaching today, a half-truth, that is Satan's specialty. We are bombarded with this philosophy in the media, magazines, and newspapers. I think we need to evaluate it in light of God's Word.

The idea is that what we are today is completely determined by what happened to us in our childhoods. In other words, our pasts control our futures. I see many examples of this type of thinking in binge eaters.

A woman came to me for counseling one day. Her hair was dirty and unkempt. She could hardly speak without breaking down in tears. Her eyes mirrored the hopelessness she felt. She had been to many counseling sessions with many counselors. She began the session by talking about her parents and her past, as I am sure she had so many times before.

I stopped her midway and asked her if she was born again. She said she was. I responded, "Mary, I want to share some things with you from the Word of God. This may be very different from what you have heard before, but it has been very important in my own life, and I believe it will help you, also."

I read to her from 2 Corinthians 5:17, *"Therefore, if anyone is in Christ, he is a new creation; old things have passed away; behold, all things have become new."* I also shared Philippians 3:13–14 with her. *"But one thing I do, forgetting those things which are behind and reaching forward to those things which are ahead, I press toward the goal for the prize of the upward call of God in Christ Jesus."* I explained to her that when she was born again, she became a new creature inside, and nothing from the past could control her future anymore.

I encouraged her to stop looking to the past for reasons for her problems, but rather to *"put on the new man which was created according to God, in true righteousness"* (Ephesians 4:24). Rather than to continually drag out the past, we are told as new creatures to *"put off, concerning your former conduct, the old man"* (v. 22). In other words, quit dragging and start pressing forward! That is what the Good News is all about. What a thrill to witness a life totally transformed by the power of Jesus Christ.

Joyful Results

She seemed surprised. She had been looking backward for so long that she had completely lost any vision for the future. Proverbs 29:18 says, *"Where there is no vision, the people perish"* (KJV). She was perishing on the inside. I told her to wash her hair, use makeup on her face, and do a number of other things during the next week. I shared with her the principles of sowing to the Spirit and showed her how this applied to her particular problem.

The next week when she came back, even I was surprised. I didn't have to ask her how she had been that week. She glowed. The entire expression of her face had changed. She met me with a smile, and her eyes were bright. What a change as she began *"forgetting those things which are behind and reaching forward to those things which are ahead"* (Philippians 3:13).

One Christian told me that she was overweight because someone had put a curse on her grandmother. Another shared that she was overweight because of her mother. Her mother had been unhappy at the prospect of having a baby, a baby who turned out to be this woman. They were allowing their pasts to determine their futures!

Stop looking for reasons for your compulsive eating. God never directed me backward—only *forward.* There was no hidden, secret reason behind my eating. I could not tell you today what caused my gluttony. But I can tell you that I am free through Christ Jesus, and I'll take that anytime!

Trials Will Come

Another easy trap to fall into is to "wait until everything settles down" for you emotionally before you try to sow to the Spirit. I can assure you now that the devil will make sure things *never* settle down if that is all it takes to keep you from victory.

Jesus tells us, *"It is impossible that no offenses should come"* (Luke 17:1). He might have added, "And they'll come often!" As one need is met, another need arises. The steadying force is knowing, *"My God shall supply all your need according to His riches in glory by Christ Jesus"* (Philippians 4:19). The peace of God that surpasses understanding is knowing that God will meet your need as you look to Him.

You are going to have situations arise in your life that cause emotional upset. Jesus said that we would have tribulation in the world (John 16:33). You can count on it. You can plan on it! But He also said, *"Be of good cheer, I have overcome the world"* (v. 33)!

My Story

In my own life, a couple of years after my healing, a situation arose that could have been disastrous to my healing. I was pregnant with our much-wanted second child when I began to bleed. The doctors told me I had only a fifty-fifty chance of carrying the baby full term. Four or five times I was put on virtual bed rest for ten days at a time. This was nothing more than a subtle scheme of the devil to try to get me back into gluttony.

He laid the trap well. This was the closest I ever came to returning to compulsive eating. But as the Word says, *"discretion will preserve you"* (Proverbs

2:11). God, through His healing, returned discretion to me—the freedom or authority to make decisions—and this discretion preserved me.

This was a time when I could have been very bored, and it was a time of emotional pressure. Both are dangerous times for former gluttons. It was a time to *"put on the whole armor of God, that* [I] *may be able to stand against the wiles of the devil"* (Ephesians 6:11). I made a choice right then to *"ponder the path of* [my] *feet, and let all* [my] *ways be established"* (Proverbs 4:26). My armor went up!

Handling the Difficulty

I planned activities for this time, *from the first day,* that led me away from eating. I determined from the first day to sow several hours of fasting each day. I made sure I would not be alone most of the time. I invited friends to visit. As always, I read my Bible and spent time in prayer each day.

I made it through with flying colors! I didn't overeat, I didn't lose the baby, and I knew from that moment forward that nothing would ever make me turn to food again—and it hasn't. That child is now married and expecting her own child. The lesson is that life isn't perfect. Things happen that we don't anticipate or understand. What we need to understand is that we are never far from His help.

Don't let anything keep you from pressing toward the mark—especially the ups and downs of daily life.

Ecclesiastes 11:4 says, *"He who observes the wind will not sow, and he who regards the clouds will not reap."* The Scripture goes on to say in verse 6, *"In the morning sow your seed."* If you are always observing your life, waiting until everything is normal to begin sowing, you will never reap. We want to wait for things to settle down and then confront our eating.

God's way is for us to first confront our eating, knowing that afterward things will settle down. We are told in Hebrews 12:1 to *"lay aside every weight, and the sin which so easily ensnares us."* Which sin? The particular sin that attacks us so easily. For a glutton or a compulsive eater, the sin is using food the wrong way. Don't try to put this problem on a back burner.

Don't Be Overwhelmed

Perhaps laying aside this sin seems absolutely overwhelming to you. If you are feeling powerless to overcome it, you are looking at *your* ability and past failures rather than to *God's* ability.

I received a letter recently from a person who was feeling overwhelmed by her problem with eating. She made a very frank and almost shocking statement. She said, "At times this obsession even supersedes God in my life." I know she was really feeling this way, but I don't believe it was really true.

I believe she just felt overwhelmed by the power that food seemed to hold over her. I believe she was trying to take on the whole problem at once, and she didn't see how in the world she could make it. I shared with her a most important principle that Jesus taught us about the kingdom of God. It is this: *"He who is faithful in what is least is faithful also in much"* (Luke 16:10). Jesus is telling us to break down that problem to the point where we can be faithful.

God Supersedes Everything

This woman desperately needed to know that God did supersede her desire for food. She needed to grow to where she could be faithful. I told her to begin tomorrow doing the following—*and nothing else*—with regard to her eating.

Take the first ten things you are tempted to eat tomorrow (other than breakfast). Hold each one in your hand when you are being tempted. Hold just that one item up and ask yourself, "Who do you love more? This Oreo cookie or Jesus?" Do the same with the next thing you are tempted to eat until you have confronted ten foods.

I know what her response will be because I have used this method often in my own life. You see, she does love the Lord more, but the devil wants us to stay overwhelmed. God wants us to start where we can, but we must start.

Sometimes we try to move a giant tree when God expects us only to plant a seed. *You do what you can, and God will do what you cannot.*

Chapter 7

Eat Whatever Is Set before You

When a person has been on many diets for many years, he is likely to make food choices that are influenced by a long list of "rights" and "wrongs." He may actually experience extreme guilt when eating certain foods because he has come to think of them as "sinful."

Some foods have come to be viewed as "good foods." If he is eating these foods, he feels that he has done well. Other foods have come to be viewed as "bad foods." If he eats these foods, he feels a self-loathing condemnation. Too much of the wrong kind of importance is given to the foods he eats.

What about what we eat? What did Jesus teach about what we eat? Food fads, or so-called "food truths," come and go, but God's Word is truth itself. There are no higher findings than what Jesus Christ taught. His life is our example in every area. It reveals truth that we can count on, truth that will last.

What Did Jesus Teach about Eating?

People today are uptight about food. There is hardly a food that isn't suspect in some circles.

Bookshelves are filled with answers about what we should and shouldn't be eating. One eats sugar; another adamantly opposes it. One eats meat; another eats only vegetables. Relationships, even among family members and brothers in the Lord, can feel the strain of the diversity of beliefs about food.

I believe Jesus was very aware of the divisions such doctrines can cause. When He sent out the seventy disciples, He gave specific instructions with regard to *what* to eat. This would have been an ideal time to give instructions and laws regarding food.

Yet His statements were simple and clear. *"And remain in the same house, eating and drinking such things as they give....Eat such things as are set before you"* (Luke 10:7–8). In other words, whatever they are eating, you eat. Eat whatever is set before you.

In Matthew 15:11, Jesus said, *"Not what goes into the mouth defiles a man; but what comes out of the mouth, this defiles a man."* What goes into the mouth? Food! Man is not defiled by what he eats.

In fact, in Matthew 6:25, Jesus tells us, *"Do not worry about your life, what you will eat or what you will drink."* This is in strong contrast to a great deal of teaching that is going forth today, even in the church. Today we hear, "Take great thought about what you are to eat."

The Spirit Speaking through Paul

Paul addressed the same subject with great consistency throughout his letters. In Colossians

2:16, he instructed us to *"let no one judge you in food or in drink."* He went on to say,

> *Therefore, if you died with Christ from the basic principles of the world, why, as though living in the world, do you subject yourselves to regulations; do not touch, do not taste.* (vv. 20–21)

Paul was unmoved by the doctrines that were coming forth, which said that people shouldn't eat certain foods.

The spiritual lesson Paul taught us was that *"food does not commend us to God; for neither if we eat are we the better, nor if we do not eat are we the worse"* (1 Corinthians 8:8). *"For the kingdom of God is not eating and drinking"* (Romans 14:17).

What about Nutrition and Health?

What about processed and non-processed foods? Some have taught that the reason Jesus was never sick was that He never ate processed foods.

Part of that is very true. Jesus did not eat processed food. *There were no processed foods at the time of Christ—yet sickness was rampant!* If not eating processed foods was the secret of good health, there should have been no sickness in Jesus' time.

Even today, in countries where there are no processed foods, the life expectancy is only half that of the United States. Nations without processed foods often face starvation and every form of sickness and disease, rather than experiencing the healthy life one would expect to find.

Importance of Processed Foods

Of course, foods can be overprocessed. The food that God designed for our bodies grows from the ground or comes from milk, meat, fish, or poultry. Some of the packaged foods have been so far removed from their original substance that they hardly qualify as food anymore. They are just packaged, processed stuff put into appealing boxes. Common sense tells you not to fill your own body or your children's bodies with something roughly equivalent to trash. That is why some things are referred to as "junk food." They are just plain junk.

Products that are artificially flavored and artificially colored with long lists of chemicals that have been added as preservatives hardly qualify as food anymore. These worthless products can bring on a "junk-funk." When this happens, it is because your body isn't getting what it needs to be strong and healthy. *Those "foods" should not be a regular part of anyone's diet!*

That doesn't mean that a person should spend an extraordinary amount of time and thought about what he eats. A simple plan is to eat what God provided. The closer it is to the way He made it, the better it will probably be for our physical bodies. Apples are a good example of the wonder of the Great Chef. They are beautifully packaged, don't need refrigeration, are easy to transport, and taste great! If you take an apple and add a few ingredients to make a delicious baked apple, you are still starting with real food.

That same apple could be squashed, strained, cooked, and mixed with so much other stuff that it is called "apple juice," but it is really only 10 or 20 percent real juice. Now it has become something other than food. It has become "junk." Don't base your eating on "junk food."

Sometimes nutritional value is needlessly lost by processing, but other times nutritional value is enhanced by it. Dried beans and dried grains are examples of foods preserved in a way that has greatly benefited mankind. Before these foods were dried, people making long journeys had to depend on what food they could find, and they often faced starvation.

The message of Scripture seems always to be balance. Don't allow food to become some rigid, legalistic bondage. It would also be foolish to use your freedom as an excuse to deprive your body of basic nutrition.

Food versus Faith

Jesus ministered to multitudes of sick people—but *He never mentioned what they were eating.*

If what we eat is so important to our health, wouldn't Jesus have mentioned it to all the sick people He dealt with? He never indicated in any way that they needed to change what they were eating.

However, He did mention faith. *"Your faith has made you well....According to your faith let it be to you....Assuredly, I say to you, I have not found such great faith, not even in Israel!"* (Matthew 9:22, 29; 8:10). He did not say, "I have not found so great a diet, not even in Israel."

Jesus ate as He instructed His disciples to do. He ate *"whatever* [was] *set before* [Him]." When walking through a cornfield—when He was hungry—He plucked corn to eat. When He passed by a fig tree—and was hungry—He reached for a fig. When He multiplied the fish and loaves, He never changed what He multiplied. He multiplied whatever was set before Him.

Some believe they should eat Ezekiel's bread (see Ezekiel 4:9). Some say we should eat as Daniel did, eating only vegetables and drinking only water. The Bible does say in Daniel 1:15 that Daniel and the children of Israel who did not eat the king's meat were *"better and fatter in flesh than all the young men who ate the portion of the king's delicacies."*

But Daniel's fairer and fatter flesh was the result of eating in *faith,* because his trust was in God. If eating vegetables and water were a health secret revealed in Scripture, then Jesus would have eaten only vegetables and water. We know that He did not.

What about Sweets?

Perhaps more than any food today, we read about sugar and sweets. Overweight people have long looked upon sweets as forbidden fruit. What about sweets? Does Scripture teach that it is wrong to eat sweets? Are they the *"deceptive food"* spoken of in Proverbs 23:3?

Actually, Scripture is filled with references to sweets, and there is a consistent pattern. When God spoke of the Promised Land, He called it a land *"flowing with milk and honey"* (Leviticus 20:24). Again, in Deuteronomy 8:8, God said He would lead them into a good land, *"a land of wheat and barley, of vines and fig trees and pomegranates, a land of olive oil and honey."*

When reading these Scriptures, keep in mind that honey is even sweeter than sugar. Honey has sixty-four calories to a tablespoon and sugar has only forty-six. Even syrups do not duplicate the sweetness of honey.

We are told that God led Moses through the wilderness, and *"He instructed him, He kept him as the apple of His eye"* (Deuteronomy 32:10). And what did He do for this man He kept *"as the apple of His eye"*? *"He made him ride in the heights of the earth, that he might eat the produce of the fields; He made him draw honey from the rock"* (v. 13). God felt sweets were important enough that He performed a miracle in order to provide honey for Moses. We are told that Moses ate the increase of the fields, so obviously, other food was available. Yet God provided *honey!*

Honey's Value

Some of the highest words of praise in Scripture have to do with sweetness. Ezekiel described the Word of God in Ezekiel 3:3, saying, *"It was in my mouth like honey in sweetness."* In Psalm 19:7, David extolled God with magnificent praises; he said, *"The law of the LORD is perfect, converting the soul; the testimony of the LORD is sure, making wise the simple."* He summed up these thoughts with, *"More to be desired are they than gold, yea, than much fine gold; sweeter also than honey and the honeycomb"* (v. 10). Would David or Ezekiel have compared the Word of God to something that was sinful or bad for us?

God's great prophet, Isaiah, prophesied, *"The Lord Himself will give you a sign: Behold, the virgin shall conceive and bear a Son, and shall call His name Immanuel"* (Isaiah 7:14). We have all read this verse with joy! It foretells the birth of our Lord. The next verse says, *"Curds and honey **He shall eat**"* (v. 15, emphasis added). We know He actually ate honey because in Luke 24:42–43, when He asked for food from the disciples, *"they gave Him a piece of a broiled fish and some honeycomb. And He took it and ate in their presence."* Again, Jesus ate exactly as He had instructed His disciples to eat. He ate whatever was set before Him.

In all Scripture, there is not a single instance where sweetness is used to mean anything but goodness. These are only a few of many examples. In fact, Proverbs 24:13 couldn't be any plainer. *"Eat honey because it is good, and the honeycomb which is sweet to your taste."* It is supposed to taste good. God went to a lot of trouble to enable you to taste sweets.

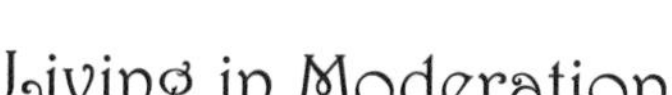

Living in Moderation

In Proverbs we are told to eat honey (sweets) because it is good and sweet to our taste. We are also cautioned, *"It is not good to eat much honey"* (Proverbs 25:27). Scripture says, *"Have you found honey? Eat only as much as you need"* (v. 16). Paul said in Philippians 4:5, *"Let your moderation be known unto all men"* (KJV).

What does that mean for us today? It means it is all right to eat sweets. God meant for you to enjoy them; but *"eat only as much as you need."* If you buy a package of six little doughnuts, and after eating two or three, you are filled, don't eat the whole package. Moderation means that if half a candy bar is sufficient for you, don't eat all of it!

Often just a taste is enough. During the time my husband lost forty-five pounds, he occasionally took doughnuts for the workers in his office. He said he was amazed to find that sometimes one-fourth of a doughnut was enough to satisfy him. Sometimes a taste is not enough to satisfy us. But learn to *"eat only as much as you need."* Don't eat what everyone else is eating, or how much is in the package, but how much is sufficient for you.

True Deceptive Food

Deceptive food, then, is not sweets; rather, it is food eaten for the wrong reasons, because of frustration, guilt, anger, or boredom. It is food eaten to help you forget your troubles rather than turn to God.

Some people have used sweets as deceptive food. They have experienced an unnatural, obsessive craving for sweets. They have eaten sweets to their condemnation so many times that they think sweets are sinful. It was the gluttonous eating of sweets that was wrong, not the sweets themselves.

If a person has a problem with lust and reads sensual books, that is wrong. But reading isn't wrong, and books aren't wrong. Being able to read is a gift from God, but it can be used the wrong way. So it is that we can use foods the wrong way, without the food itself being wrong.

We have looked at sugar, or honey, from a scriptural standpoint because that is the view that will stand. Even in the medical community there is no agreement about sugar being bad. The following information comes from "Medical Q & A," a medical column written by Dr. Neil Solomon and carried in newspapers all over the country.

Medical View of Sugar

A gentleman had written in because his wife was trying to get him to stop using sugar. He asked Dr. Solomon:

"If I am wrong about the use of sugar, in what is an otherwise sound diet, I'd like to be told about it."

Here are some excerpts from his reply:

"I can say *there is little to suggest* that the use of sugar contributes significantly to cardiovascular disease, diabetes, or surprisingly, obesity." (It should not surprise us since God's Word says sweets are all right, but obesity is not.)

He went on to cite a study by Dr. Frank Nuttall that showed, "Even though sugar consumption in the United States has either remained the same or increased slightly since 1968, deaths from coronary heart disease have decreased. Similarly, death from coronary heart disease is low in Cuba, Venezuela, and Colombia, even though sugar consumption in these countries is very high.

"As for development of diabetes, the primary determining factor in the case of adults is *obesity, not sugar consumption.*"

Direction for Today

What we are seeing today is a fulfillment of the prophecy given by Paul in 1 Timothy 4:1, 3–4,

> *Now the Spirit expressly says that in latter times some will depart from the faith, giving heed to deceiving spirits and doctrines of demons,... forbidding to marry, and commanding to abstain from foods which God created to be received with thanksgiving by those who believe and know the truth. For every creature of God is good, and nothing is to be refused if it is received with thanksgiving.*

These two teachings—forbidding to marry, and abstaining from certain foods—*have gained acceptance in the secular world.* The idea of living together without the covenant relationship of marriage is hardly noticed in many circles. Among this same group are many who believe it is wrong to eat meat.

Paul went on to say, *"If you instruct the brethren in these things, you will be a good minister of Jesus Christ"* (1 Timothy 4:6). So let me say it again—*food is not sinful—overeating is.* It is not wrong to eat meat; it is not wrong to eat sugar; it is not wrong to eat non-organic foods; it is not wrong to eat processed foods.

Conversely, it is not holy to eat organic foods. It is not holy to abstain from sugar. It is not holy to abstain from meat.

Natural Desires for Healthful Foods

This is not to say that nutrition has no place in our lives, but that we are not to build our lives around it. As a person begins to eat from real hunger, he has a natural desire for healthier foods.

To illustrate this, picture yourself on a camping trip. One day you decide to climb a big hill by the camp area. You begin early, and it takes a long time to get to the top. Every once in a while you stop to rest, and then you continue your climb. It is a beautiful, clear day. At the top, the view is breathtaking, and you spend quite a while admiring it.

As you start down the hill, it is evening, and you realize you haven't eaten all day. When you finally get back to camp, you are really hungry. On one side are cookies, candy bars, and potato chips.

On the other side is a pan with fresh fish frying, corn on the cob, and maybe some fresh tomatoes. Which foods would you choose? Of course, the universal response is to choose the fish and corn.

This helps to illustrate our *natural desire* for healthier foods when we eat only from real hunger. It is all part of the perfect God-given hunger response.

Deprived Childhood

Dr. William Slonecker, the well-known pediatrician from Nashville, Tennessee, had this to say about children who have eating problems: "The problem is that we do not let that child get hungry. Any child who has never been hungry, I feel, is a deprived child. He needs to be hungry enough to know what good, solid food tastes like."

My youngest daughter had a friend who had eaten nothing but "health foods" all her life. She never even tasted a cookie until she was three years old. That was because she ate one at nursery school. Her mother drove all over town to find organic foods. They never used sugar.

They did everything "right" as far as nutrition was concerned, but that child was always sick! She was always getting a cold, fever, or whatever was going around. My daughter was almost never sick, and we ate all things in moderation. Sickness comes from Satan, and *"the weapons of our warfare are not carnal but mighty in God"* (2 Corinthians 10:4).

Your Source of Strength

Our strength and our health come from God. We are told in Isaiah 40:31, *"Those who wait on the* LORD *shall renew their strength; they shall mount up with wings like eagles, they shall run and not be weary, they shall walk and not faint."*

Paul said in 1 Timothy 4:8, *"Bodily exercise profits a little, but godliness is profitable for all things." Godliness* is profitable to our bodies! Proverbs doesn't tell us, "Attend to your diet; do not let concern about what you eat depart from your eyes, for it is health to all your flesh." Rather, it says,

> *My son, give attention to my words; incline your ear to my sayings. Do not let them* [God's words] *depart from your eyes; keep them* [God's words] *in the midst of your heart; for they* [God's words] *are life to those who find them, and health to all their flesh.* (Proverbs 4:20–22)

I have seen people who are just as obsessed with *what* they eat as gluttons are about *how much* they eat. Some of the most ungodly people I know eat nothing but health foods and exercise constantly. Their *bodies* have become their top priority.

There are also some very godly people who eat nothing but health foods, and that is fine. The point is that it doesn't matter what you eat as long as food and eating keep their proper place in your life.

Why Is This Freedom Important to Know?

It is important to have this freedom with regard to what we eat. If you think certain foods are sinful, Satan will heap condemnation upon you each time you eat them. If you eat a candy bar, he will say, "Well, you know you shouldn't have eaten that. Now you have blown it. You might as well go ahead and gorge now." Condemnation over eating that one candy bar will cause you to eat three other candy bars, two doughnuts, and all of last night's leftovers!

Conversely, when you see from God's Word that it is not wrong to eat that candy bar, but that you should *"eat only as much as you need"* (Proverbs 25:16), you will begin to eat smaller portions of a big candy bar. Without condemnation over eating a chocolate, you will begin to eat one or two instead of half the box. You will begin to cut yourself small pieces of pie because you will no longer feel you must *"eat, drink, and be merry"* (Luke 12:19) because tomorrow you may diet. Rather, you will know that if you want more tomorrow, it will be all right to eat more.

Freedom in Action

I recently saw this principle beautifully illustrated. I was having lunch with a woman who lost over fifty pounds by making the changes she read about in this book. We had a lovely lunch, and afterward the waiter brought us an elegant dessert menu. The menu listed crepes filled with whipped cream and covered with fresh strawberries or a special praline sauce. We both felt totally free to order any dessert on the menu. But we had already eaten *"as much as* [we] *need*[ed]." We decided not to eat dessert.

We made this choice in total freedom. It was different from when we were compulsive eaters. If we had ordered the dessert before we were healed, we would have felt tremendous condemnation. Guilt would have led us to continue eating all day because we had "already blown it for today."

If we had *not* ordered the dessert, but still wanted it, we would have thought about that dessert for the rest of the day. We might have even eaten other foods trying to satisfy that desire. Being free to eat all things, it was a simple decision. There would have been no condemnation if we had ordered it, and there was no lingering desire when we did not. *That's freedom, and it's wonderful.*

Why Are You Eating?

It is not *what* you eat but *why* you eat that is important to God. You can sinfully overeat carrot sticks. You can sinfully overeat celery. You can sinfully overeat any food. In Psalm 78:27–31, we see this concept illustrated. *"He also rained meat on them like the dust, feathered fowl like the sand of the seas"* (v. 27).

Now there was certainly nothing wrong with the quails, since God Himself provided them. But as we read on, we are told,

> *So they ate and were well filled* [not "filled" but "well filled"], *for He gave them their own desire. They were not deprived of their craving* [for food]; *but while their food was still in their mouths, the wrath of God came against them,...and struck down the choice men of Israel.* (vv. 29–31)

It was not what they ate, but why they ate.

Romans 14:20 says, *"All things indeed are pure, but it is evil for the man who eats with offense."* If after reading these Scriptures you do not yet have total freedom to eat all things, don't eat them. Scripture says,

> *For one believes he may eat all things, but he who is weak eats only vegetables. Let not him who eats despise him who does not eat, and let not him who does not eat judge him who eats.* (Romans 14:2–3)

I believe that as you study God's Word you will come to have this freedom. But until you do, don't go against your conscience.

Convictions about Food

Some people feel a conviction that they shouldn't eat certain foods. I once heard a pastor friend tell about a very precious friend who didn't eat pork. When they ate together, his friend merely said, "Brother, I feel a conviction that I should not have pork."

The pastor respected this, although he felt no such conviction. Neither tried to persuade the other of the "error of his thinking," but lived the

Scripture, *"Let not him who does not eat judge him who eats."*

God never desires that individual convictions about food or drink divide His body. The question is, "Who is Lord of your life?"

Jesus reminds us in Matthew 11:18–19, *"For John came neither eating nor drinking, and they say, 'He has a demon.' The Son of Man came eating and drinking, and they say, 'Look, a glutton and a winebibber.'"* At one point Jesus said, *"Among those born of women there has not risen one greater than John the Baptist"* (v. 11). Yet He ate exactly the opposite of what John ate.

During the time of my healing, there were certain foods that I knew I consistently tended to overeat. I avoided these foods as seed to the Spirit and as a way of choosing God in my eating. Now I can eat all foods with complete freedom. But start where you are.

People can get so caught up in eating or not eating certain foods that they miss the whole point: *Jesus is the answer*—not what foods we eat or don't eat. Our bodies are not sanctified by the food we eat; rather our food is sanctified by the Word of God and prayer. (See 1 Timothy 4:4–5.)

Chapter 8

Giving Thanks

When we think of saying grace before we eat, we often have a mental picture of a Norman Rockwell-type family. They are sitting around the table at Sunday dinner, heads bowed and eyes closed. The children are peeking or secretly feeding the dog their Brussels sprouts. Sweet and serene families are gathered together.

But when Jesus gave thanks to God for His food, things happened! When He thanked God for the five loaves and two fish, they were multiplied to feed over five thousand men, women, and children, with twelve baskets of food left over!

> *He took the five loaves and the two fish, and looking up to heaven, He blessed and broke and gave the loaves to the disciples; and the disciples gave to the multitudes. So they all ate.* (Matthew 14:19–20)

Again, in Matthew 15:36–37, we read that as Jesus took the seven loaves and fish and gave thanks, they were multiplied to feed four thousand men, plus women and children. *"And He took the seven loaves and the fish and gave thanks, broke them and gave them to His disciples; and the disciples gave to the multitude. So they all ate."* After Jesus' resurrection, it was at the precise moment when He blessed the bread that the disciples' eyes were opened to know Him.

> *Now it came to pass, as He sat at the table with them, that He took bread, blessed and broke it, and gave it to them. Then their eyes were opened and they knew Him; and He vanished from their sight.*
> (Luke 24:30–31)

Releasing Supernatural Power

There was a release of supernatural power when Jesus thanked God for His food. Paul said in 1 Timothy 4:4–5, *"Nothing is to be refused if it is received with thanksgiving; for it is sanctified by the word of God and prayer." Sanctified* means "purified, made conducive to spiritual blessing, freed from sin."

While Jesus placed little emphasis on *what* He ate, He placed great emphasis on *praying* over His food, thanking God for what He was about to eat. One of the things we teach in our Scriptural Eating Classes is the importance of thanking God for our food. A person who is seeking victory with his eating should thank God every time he begins to eat anything.

Least Likely to Say Grace

Have you ever noticed how often a person thanks God for his food while on a binge? *Never!*

When a person is alone, that is the time he is the *least* likely to thank God for his food and ask God's blessing on it. But that is the most important time.

When we head to the kitchen for a "little snack," that is another time we are unlikely to say grace over our food. Yet that is the time we are most likely to eat to our condemnation—to sinfully overeat.

During the time of my healing, God led me to pray over everything I ate. I don't mean that I prayed over each bite of food during a meal, but I do mean that I prayed *every time* I started to eat. I still remember the prayer after all these years. "Father, I pray that You will bless this food to the strength and nourishment of my body, that it might not serve as condemnation, that I might not hate others or myself."

Praying before you eat is especially important when you are alone. Often just the act of thanking God for the food you are about to eat is enough to stop you from eating it. It is impossible to sincerely thank God for food you know you should not be eating. *I have never known a glutton who consistently prayed over everything he ate.*

I recently received a letter from a woman in South Africa that illustrates this "sanctification" principle that Paul spoke of and Jesus illustrated by example. She was so impressed with the results of learning to give thanks for everything she was eating that she wrote this letter:

"I am writing to thank you for the teaching on *Least Likely to Say Grace.* I just came from school.

Normally I make myself a cup of tea, and go for my snack. I just had this nice, big sweet roll. (Sound familiar?)" She was getting ready to eat in a way that would probably lead to trouble for her; she was tired and alone.

A statement from the book rose up inside of her, "When is a person least likely to thank God for his food?" She stopped, prayed, and received *immediate help.* She didn't even want to eat it after that!

She made a spiritual decision that changed her physical circumstances, and the results were powerful and, in this case, immediate.

We cannot see, touch, taste, or smell supernatural things. They are spiritual, and our spirit does not operate with physical senses. That is why we accept some things "on faith." She remembered the example of Jesus, believed what she had read, acted on it by stopping to pray, and received help that would not have been there any other way.

What Jesus illustrated about giving thanks for our food must be understood through faith. If you don't believe it, you won't do it.

Praying before Temptation Arrives

Peter learned a bitter lesson about the power of prayer *before* you enter into temptation. Jesus prayed the night before He was betrayed. He told Peter he would deny Him, but Peter was full of confidence. *"Even if all are made to stumble because of You, I will never be made to stumble"* (Matthew 26:33). Peter meant this with all his heart as he was saying it.

Later, as Jesus prepared Himself through prayer for His coming trial, Peter fell asleep. Jesus woke Peter and told him, *"Watch and pray, lest you enter into temptation. The spirit indeed is willing, but the flesh is weak"* (Matthew 26:41). Jesus was telling Peter that if he would take the time to prepare himself spiritually through prayer, he would not have to give in to the temptation that would later break Peter's heart. Conversely, Jesus was warning him that if he did not pray, he would enter into temptation and fall because the flesh is weak. Peter's good intentions were not enough to see him through this temptation.

Strengthening Your Good Intentions

I see much correlation between this episode and people caught in any compulsive sin. How many times they go to sleep confident that "tomorrow I am going to do better." Like Peter, we all have good intentions. We mean it with all our hearts. We don't intend to fall, but we are still trusting in our flesh, which is weak.

The Bible says that Peter *"wept bitterly"* (Matthew 26:75; Luke 22:62). He was angry with himself and full of condemnation. He cried bitter tears of regret. This is a familiar pattern to a person caught in compulsive sin. Jesus said Peter could have been spared falling into this temptation if he had taken the time to prepare himself through prayer, *beforehand.*

"Watch and pray, lest you enter into temptation" (Matthew 26:41). Watch—be alert to the danger.

Plan out your day with non-eating activities. And pray—pray before you enter into temptation. Peter's prayers would have made the difference for him, and your prayers will make the difference in your being able to stand.

Chapter 9
A Plan to Last a Lifetime

Now that I have been free from binge eating or gluttony for over twenty years, I still observe the two-meal-a-day eating pattern most of the time. This eating pattern has proved itself for me through the years. It was not the source of my healing, but rather just a better way of eating that I discovered. I would never want to go back to eating three regular meals a day. Something very positive would be missing from my life.

I do, however, allow myself more freedom to eat snacks. I don't hesitate to eat an ice cream cone with the kids or coffee cake with a friend. It is a beautiful thing to be able to eat these things without condemnation, to know it will not bring on a binge. I thank God for freedom from that nagging urge to eat.

I also have lunch when a friend invites me. If I have a luncheon meeting, I go, eat lunch, and thoroughly enjoy it! There is certainly no condemnation when I eat lunch. I just don't eat three meals a day on a consistent basis.

Hunger by Suggestion

I have found that if I know I am going to be eating lunch, I will actually be hungry by lunchtime; whereas if I know I am not going to eat lunch that day, I will not be hungry. That is why it is important to *purpose in your heart* when you are going to observe the lunch fast or dinner fast. Simply tell your body when you wake up that morning, "This is how it is going to be!"

One of the reasons I feel this has been such a satisfactory plan for all these years—and will continue to be for the rest of my life—is that *I never give up the foods I enjoy when I eat.* Again, let me repeat that dieting is not mentioned in Scripture, but fasting is. For we are dead

> *with Christ from the basic principles of the world* [and commandments and doctrines of men that say],...*"Do not touch, do not taste, do not handle," which all concern things which perish with the using....*[But rather we] *set* [our] *mind* [focus of our life] *on things above, not on things on the earth* [constant concern about what we are going to eat, when we are going to eat, how much we are going to eat].
>
> (Colossians 2:20; 3:2)

Forty-Something Living

Our bodies change in many ways through the years. One change is that we tend to use fewer and fewer calories as we grow older. A person can steadily gain weight without changing what he is eating. The weight gain may be so gradual that you hardly notice it until you have gone up a dress or suit size or two. If someone is gaining only two pounds a year, at the end of ten years he will have put on twenty additional pounds.

I realized that I was gradually gaining weight, but I wasn't eating any more than I had been. In fact, I didn't feel it would be healthy to eat less, since I wasn't overeating at all. I went back to the One who set me free. I asked for help, and He gave it.

If you find you are gradually gaining weight, here are some things that I have found that have helped me to maintain my weight and my health, as well.

Exercise

You have to do a whole lot of exercise to lose weight, but you don't have to do a whole lot of exercise to help maintain weight and health. This is because the benefit of exercise continues long after you have stopped exercising. Exercise builds muscle to replace fat, and muscle burns one-third more calories than fat. Just by building up more muscle, you can eat more without gaining weight.

Another benefit that continues after exercising is the increase in metabolism. This continues for several hours after vigorous exercise and causes your body to use more calories. Rushing blood flow and perspiration are both healthy body functions that increase during and after exercise.

In fact, exercise is probably one of the healthiest life choices that you can make. How effective is it in maintaining overall health? It is quite dramatic. People who do vigorous exercise for twenty minutes a day, three times a week, are 50 percent less likely to get all diseases—50 percent less cancer, 50 percent less diabetes, 50 percent less heart disease, 50 percent less flu, 50 percent fewer strokes, 50 percent fewer colds!

It seemed like an impressive statistic when I heard it a number of years ago. For me, it was part of the "answer" that I had asked God for. As soon as I heard it, my spirit bore witness with it, and I knew that I was being given the wisdom I had asked for. I began to incorporate that relatively small amount of vigorous exercise into my life from the time I heard of its benefits.

My experience would certainly back up what I had heard. I haven't been to a doctor for sickness in seven years. I have heard it said, "If exercise was a medicine, it would be the most prescribed drug in the world."

Exercise has additional benefits, as well. It helps maintain muscle tone, physical strength, flexibility, and emotional stability. It keeps joints moving. After forty, many people experience "frozen joints" because of lack of use. It is very painful and can require surgery. Our bodies were meant to move, bend, and reach. All the remotes in our lives invite us to a lifestyle that is greatly diminished physically. That extremely sedentary lifestyle will exact a price later on. We have all the remotes that anyone could want, but my husband and I both make sure that we also keep our bodies moving. You can save yourself a lot of health problems by choosing to exercise.

What kinds of exercise? Find something you love, and do it! I know people in their sixties who are kick-boxing. Some people do well with indoor, year-round swimming. You may prefer group exercise and find the stimulation and encouragement of others to be important.

Almost anyone can go for a twenty-minute walk, and being outside seems to be a good choice for people who tend toward melancholy. The weather does not need to restrict your walking if you are dressed for it, with the one exception of ice. Don and I have taken some of our most memorable long walks in very cold weather with lots of warm layers. It takes somewhere in the vicinity of twenty minutes. Treadmills can provide an easy and safe way to exercise at home. Ski machines give an excellent and very vigorous workout. There are many helpful exercise videos that can be used. Even if you have some physical limitations, a good physical therapist can show you ways to exercise around your limitations.

After forty, both men and women should do some weight lifting or resistance training to maintain strength. Muscle strength will diminish if it isn't challenged, and that can result in injuries. "Use it or lose it" is the rule of muscles. A person never loses the ability to build up muscle strength. That may seem strange, but your bones will thank you for it. Resistance training, or weight lifting, helps maintain bone density. It also takes years off your appearance. Stationary weight machines are an excellent choice for both men and women. They help maintain muscle strength, and that helps prevent those painful joint and back injuries.

Incorporating twenty minutes of vigorous exercise three times a week is just a smart thing to do. You will feel better and look better. You will be healthier. The only downside to it is that it takes effort to get started. I cannot honestly say that I look forward to my exercise, but I have no doubt at all of the long-term benefits. JUST DO IT. I want you to feel better and live longer.

Drink More Water

Almost anyone can benefit from drinking lots more water. This may be one of the healthiest trends that has come up in many years. Drinking lots of water every day will make you healthier. There is something about water that is different than anything else you can drink. People who are working hard—young or old—have a strong preference for water.

Drinking lots more water was a healthy choice I made for my life. My husband observed with astonishment that I would pay "good money" for water over a soda! For a number of years, I couldn't convince him to give it a try. Then about six months ago, he drastically increased his water intake and also experienced several wonderful, beneficial changes in his health.

He is an engineer, and I am certainly not a physician, but I know the benefit that we have both experienced with this very simple change in our lifestyle. Another side benefit is that it helps to keep that gradual weight gain from becoming a problem. Bottled water really does taste good, and even my husband now believes it is a good investment!

Learn a Little about Fats

Watching your fat intake just makes good sense. Develop a habit of looking at the fat content of foods that are packaged. You don't have to worry about the food God made—by that I mean fruits, vegetables, whole grains, and reasonable servings of meats, fish, or eggs. They are never overloaded with fats like a lot of packaged foods are. You don't need that extra fat anytime in your life, but after forty, it can be the culprit that is causing you additional weight gain.

Balance and Moderation

Those two words may sound boring, but they are the pavement stones of the road to Life. Jesus lived a life that focused on the big issues and always kept other things in balance. Jesus ate and enjoyed His food. That is one of the wonderful benefits of being freed from binge eating or any other obsession or habit. You can enjoy food in a way that was never possible before.

We have some precious friends who are going to Mexico as missionaries, and *what* they are going to eat is the furthest thing from their minds and hearts. They are going to bring God's Word to lost people. They have *"set* [their] *mind on things above"* (Colossians 3:2). God is their Source.

When Jesus had fasted for forty days and forty nights, Satan came to tempt Him with food, saying, *"If You are the Son of God, command this stone to become bread"* (Luke 4:3). Today he says, "You can't go without food! You'll ruin your health. Think of your protein! Think of your vitamins!"

"But Jesus answered him, saying, 'It is written, "Man shall not live by bread alone, but by every word of God"'" (v. 4).

God's Word is the answer. We see in later Scriptures where Jesus ate and enjoyed His food. He ate as He instructed His disciples to eat, *"such things as are set before you"* (Luke 10:8), but His priorities were right.

Some Benefits of Eating Two Meals

I have found that if I have gained a few extra pounds on vacation or over a holiday (and you will from time to time), I actually look forward to getting back to a schedule of two meals a day. I miss being hungry when I eat! Almost everyone has, at some point, experienced a time when they were not able to eat and were quite hungry when they finally ate.

The food just seemed to taste extra good. I have had similar comments from others who have tried eating only two meals a day. They are amazed at how easily their bodies adapt, and how good their food tastes.

If you are in the weight-losing phase, and you are not losing as fast as you would like, cut back some on the amount you eat for both of your meals. It's easy to kid yourself about how much you're eating, but the scales won't lie! Do not start restricting what you eat, *only how much you eat.* Don't get back in the "lettuce and tomato" syndrome. Go ahead and eat the foods you enjoy, but eat somewhat less until you find the amount you can eat and still lose weight.

Lifetime Habits

Remember, we are talking about a lifetime change in your eating habits. If you restrict yourself from the foods you enjoy, you will not want to cut back on your eating after a holiday, for example. Just be *faithful* with the fasting you offer to God. It's fine to start small; just be sure you start faithful. *"He who is faithful in what is least is faithful also in much"* (Luke 16:10). Be faithful in your daily fasting, and you will also be faithful in the larger things (weight loss).

I have found victory in many other areas of my life by using God's Word and sowing to the Spirit rather than to the flesh. Not long ago I was visiting with a young woman I had known for many years. She told me something that I didn't know before. She had never had a weight problem, but she had heard me teach one time about sowing to the Spirit. She said, "Diane, I have used those principles many times in my life and in many areas. They really changed my life." Wow!

My healing from gluttony was the beginning of my realization of who Jesus is, and what He really did for us. I will always have a special place in my heart for overweight people because I have been there. I know what it feels like inside. But now I am thin, and I know what that feels like, too. I thank God for the freedom that He purchased for us through His own Son Jesus.

Chapter 10

Seven Roadblocks to Total Healing

I have seen people in our classes begin in great victory. Their faces glow with spiritual illumination, but occasionally that glow begins to fade. I have found there are seven areas where it is easy to fall. If you are not experiencing all the success you feel you should be, check yourself in these seven areas:

1. *Trying to take on the whole problem at once instead of taking one day at a time as Jesus instructed.* (See Matthew 6:34.) We are given the grace, the strength, and the power to live in total victory this day. Don't try to take on the whole problem at once. One woman shared that for over a month after coming to class, she had no weight loss. She said that each week after class she would think, "Tomorrow I am going to fast for two or three days." And each week she would not even make it home without eating. The next week she would again get stirred up and decide, "Tomorrow I am really going to fast."

Finally, she decided to take only that day. She resolved in her heart to be faithful until she got home after class. The next day, she determined not to eat between meals, and to offer the fasting to

God. Before long, she was fasting one entire meal and losing weight. This change came because she started by taking one day at a time.

2. *Getting back into the "diet syndrome," restricting yourself from certain foods.* The diet syndrome says, "I've already had pancakes for breakfast. I might as well eat today." A woman called to ask for prayer. I prayed with her and suggested that she determine in her heart what seed she was going to sow to the Spirit when we hung up the phone. She said, "I've already eaten some candy—I guess I'll have to wait until tomorrow." Since this is not a diet, you have never blown it for the day! *"For a righteous man may fall seven times and rise again"* (Proverbs 24:16). Simply rise up again! Start sowing to the Spirit from that moment.

3. *Knowingly sowing to the flesh.* (See Galatians 6:7 and Romans 6:16.) Before you read this book, you may not have realized there were certain times and activities when you consistently tended to overeat. Each time you now choose such an activity, you are sowing to the flesh. If you continue to sow to the flesh, you will continue to reap from the flesh. Resist the devil. Move into non-eating activities.

4. *Leaving your house empty.* (See Matthew 12:43.) Jesus tells us that when the unclean spirit is gone out of a man (the spirit of overeating), it looks for another place to live. But if it can't find one, it returns. If the house is empty (for example, he is still watching TV when he knows it leads to overeating), it brings seven other spirits more

wicked than itself (Mr. Binge, Mr. Condemnation, Mr. Depression, and so on). You cannot stand on God's Word without a foundation. Don't leave your house empty—fill yourself with God's Word. You can't stand on God's Word if you don't *know* God's Word. Find Scriptures to help you not to worry or feel other negative emotions.

5. *Sowing from your abundance rather than from your want.* (See Mark 12:44.) What was sowing from your want last week may not be sowing from your want this week. You know when you are sowing from your want, and God knows when you are sowing from your want. Sowing from your want is not skipping a meal that you normally skip. It is not working through your lunch hour when the boss tells you to work through your lunch hour. *Sowing from your want is what you give up for Jesus' sake and the Gospel's.* (See Mark 10:29.)

6. *Sowing in a hit-or-miss manner.* (See 2 Corinthians 9:6.) We are told in this passage that he who *"sows sparingly will also reap sparingly."* If you sow to the Spirit one day and not the next, if you fast on Monday and eat Tuesday through Thursday, then maybe try fasting on Friday, you will reap the same kind of sporadic help. If you sow sparingly (hit-or-miss commitment), you will also reap sparingly (hit-or-miss help).

7. *Not being faithful with the seed you have decided to sow.* (See Luke 16:10.) Don't take on more than you can handle. Start where you are. Don't be afraid to start small—but start faithfully. Humanly, we want to start big, but Jesus said to start small.

In Matthew 13:31, He compared the kingdom of heaven to a tiny mustard seed:

> *The kingdom of heaven* [with regard to gluttony] *is like a mustard seed* [small seeds sown to the Spirit from your want], *which a man took and sowed in his field* [your life], *which indeed is the least of all the seeds* [biggest problem in your life—overeating—taken care of]; *but when it is grown it is greater than the herbs and becomes a tree, so that the birds of the air come and nest in its branches* [you will be a witness and blessing to others who have the same problem].

You don't have to ask yourself, "Is this going to work?" God's Word works 100 percent of the time. You can be free for the rest of your life in Jesus' name.

That freedom is what Jesus Christ, the Savior of the world, the sacrificial Lamb, the Son of Man, is all about.

Chapter 11

A Man's Perspective by Don Hampton

I had spent the first thirty-seven years of my life being basically overweight. Not always fat, but never slim. I began battling hypertension, or high blood pressure, at the age of fifteen. I never really attempted to maintain my weight. I was active and always tall for my age.

In my younger years, I thought I was ten or fifteen pounds overweight. In reality, the scales showed I was over twenty pounds too heavy. As the years crept by, and my lifestyle became more sedentary, the scales began creeping constantly upward.

The gain was consistent but slow. I would occasionally try one of Diane's many new "fad" diets. Yuck! I still remember the banana and milk diet. I didn't care much for bananas to begin with. That was over twenty years ago, and I still cringe when I pass a bunch of bananas in the store.

Naturally, none of the diets had a lasting effect. I still preferred my double serving of chili, hot dogs, or Mexican food. Sometime in my early thirties, I unconsciously decided not to actively fight my weight anymore. Life was easier at that point because the frustration caused by dieting was gone. But the excess weight continued to silently do its deadly damage. My weight rose from 220 to 230, 235, and finally to over 240 pounds.

Kidding Myself

Boy, was I oblivious to my own surroundings! Diane's weight was well under control. She hadn't been on any silly diets for eight or ten years. She was much happier. I didn't find her crying about her weight anymore. She really looked super and had looked great for years.

She talked about how God had healed her of compulsive eating, and I thought, "Great!" But it didn't make much sense to me. Besides, I didn't look so bad at 240 pounds! Since my awakening, it amazes me how overweight people deceive themselves.

After having maintained her weight for ten years, Diane had an opportunity to share her experience. We expected a small group of about half-a-dozen ladies. That group of six was closer to fifty, and it grew to over one hundred men and women. The group continued to meet for about nine months! Sometimes Diane taught three different classes each week. People were hungry to hear what God could do in this area.

After our pastor reviewed the class materials, he asked Diane if she had ever considered writing a book. Diane also felt the class needed something written to enable them to grasp these concepts better. Also, she was receiving many invitations to speak, and she was physically unable to meet all the demands herself. With my encouragement, she began writing. This was the birth of Scriptural Living Ministries and Diane's first book. You are reading an expanded, revised version of the original book, *Scriptural Eating Patterns.*

A Witness to His Wonders

As a faithful and loving husband, I began proofreading and critiquing each page. I am positive that I must have read the original book at least thirty-two times before we decided it was ready to print. Let me tell you this; after reading a book thirty-two times, you *know* what the book is about! I decided, along with a little encouragement from the Lord, that maybe I wasn't a good witness being overweight.

I began putting God's principles about weight and eating to use in my life. I immediately discovered that following them exactly as set forth in the book did not fit my schedule as a businessman. I often spent the lunch hour with clients. I wasn't going to tell my client, "I am fasting, but go ahead and enjoy a nice meal." No way. Still, the principles made sense to me.

Being quick to learn (after all, it took me only eleven years and thirty-two times through the book to figure out why Diane remains slim and trim), I made a slight modification to the program.

Breakfast was out. I ate a normal, enjoyable lunch, and, for most of the next three months, I skipped dinner.

I never stopped eating the foods I enjoyed. I still ate chili and Mexican food, but I considered my full response. I ordered only one double chili burger instead of two. I even got to the point where I didn't even order a double. The whole program fit in well with my schedule as a businessman.

Three months, forty-five pounds, and six inches off the waist later, I was amazed to see that the excess weight was gone forever. That was almost twenty years ago. A couple of years later, during a period of heavy stress, I began to let go of the principles, and I gained weight. I reapplied God's Word, however, and my body came right back into subjection to me.

Blood Pressure Miracle

Two amazing—really miraculous—things occurred as I applied God's Word. Of course, I lost weight, but my high blood pressure (essentially hypertension, which is considered incurable) began to drop into the normal range for the first time in twenty years! The doctor had no explanation for this. So I gave him one of Diane's books. I give the glory to God. Diets never affected my blood pressure, but the principles in God's Word did.

The second thing is that for the first time in my life, I am not under bondage to eat at a certain time. Before, if I was even late for a meal, I was shaky, sick, and irritable. Believe me, I *never* missed a meal! Now I can go all day without eating, if necessary. Sometimes I get into a business meeting where we need to work through the lunch hour. Now, it is no problem for me.

Not Always Easy

Sometimes I would teach the last class of a series, and I always pointed out that the weight-loss period was not always easy for me. There were times when I was hungry. I was surprised to find that this hunger was often more easily satisfied than I ever dreamed possible.

Sometimes doughnuts or fresh cookies would show up at the office. The temptation for a taste would really get to me. I defeated this by saying, "Okay, taste buds, you want a taste? That's all you are going to have." That one taste was enough for me, and it satisfied that driving urge to eat. Eventually, I was able to bypass even that small sample.

I praise God and thank Him for raising up Diane to teach Scriptural Eating Patterns. I know, that, through a healthier body, God has given me a new lease on life. As you complete this book, my prayers are with you. I pray that you will have the courage to make a commitment that will enable God to give you a new lease on life.

Commonly Asked Questions

Question: I am a diabetic. What about me?

Answer: In every situation, there is always a way to sow to the Spirit. Obviously, you did not become overweight by following the diabetic diet. Look at the times you have the most problems with eating and begin sowing those times to the Spirit. Also, you could simply purpose in your heart to follow the diet your doctor gave you. Offer that to God as seed to the Spirit. *Do what you can do, and God will do what you cannot do.*

Question: Is it safe to eat two meals when you are pregnant?

Answer: Yes! First, let's look at your question scripturally. God Himself would feed His creation correctly. Therefore, we can see how He provided for pregnant women in Scripture.

In Exodus 16:12, we see the Lord providing for the children of Israel in the desert. He said, *"At twilight* [in the evening] *you shall eat meat, and in the morning you shall be filled with bread."* Two meals, morning and evening. We know, if we read further, that this food was provided in such a way that it would be impossible to eat more often. In the morning, as the sun's heat increased, the food melted. If the Israelites tried to keep the manna overnight, it bred worms and began to stink.

We *know* that many of these women were pregnant because a whole generation was born in the wilderness. God made no special provision for the pregnant women. We can see that two meals a day is scripturally sound for pregnant women.

In my own experience, I had no trouble observing a two-meal-a-day eating pattern during pregnancy. I did, however, drink a glass of milk or eat an occasional small snack if I felt hungry. As always, I found this eating pattern was a vital key to maintaining my weight. I gained exactly what the doctor suggested with both pregnancies. And I lost all the extra weight within a few months after giving birth. Both of our babies were fat and healthy—8 pounds and 7 ½ pounds!

Question: When you are fasting, are drinks allowed?

Answer: Absolutely! The only exception would be if you have a real problem drinking too much. I drank coffee with cream, and one soda or a glass of fruit juice in the afternoon—but only if I desired it. Don't make fasting too hard on yourself! We are sowing *control* with our eating—not a complete fast. We are looking for lifetime changes in our eating patterns. Total fasting could hardly become a lifetime eating pattern.

Question: How do you feel about diet foods?

Answer: For the most part, I believe it is a mistake to use diet products. They tend to promote the thinking, "It is *always* all right to eat this because it is low in calories"; or the idea, "I can eat all I want because it is low-calorie." You are not relearning your God-given hungry and full responses.

I also believe that diet foods have a much lower ability to satisfy. I never used any diet products during the time of my weight loss. It was a joy to be able to eat "real food" without condemnation for the first time. And I found it much more satisfying.

Question: I have over one hundred pounds to lose. Will these principles work for me?

Answer: Yes and no. Yes, healing is available; and no, I do not feel that fasting one meal a day will meet your total need. The greatest success seems to come by cutting down to *one meal* a day. Almost every person who has had over one hundred pounds to lose has told me they find it just as easy to cut back to one meal.

Also, increase your vegetable intake with your meal. Many people with over one hundred pounds to lose don't eat any vegetables at all! This is far from the "moderation" that Scripture teaches. God can change your desire for certain foods! Believe God for a change in the foods you really enjoy.

If your budget has been tight, and you have leaned toward starchy menus because of this, you will be able to afford meats you could not afford before. When you eliminate one or two meals a day, you will see quite a savings at the grocery store. One lady told me, "I was actually shocked to realize how much I was spending on food." One couple said they were able to afford steaks for the first time in their marriage! This doesn't mean you should cut out all starches. But avoid meals that use starches, such as macaroni and cheese, as a main dish. Eat all things, but in moderation.

Question: I've had some real emotional upsets and a lot on my mind lately. Shouldn't I wait until things settle down before I try to deal with my eating?

Answer: Absolutely not! Emotional upsets and mental stress are greatly exaggerated and magnified by overeating. The Bible says, *"'Bread eaten in secret is pleasant.' But...her guests are in the depths of hell"* (Proverbs 9:17–18). During such a time, you need something that is going to lift you up, not something that is going to drag you down to the depths of hell.

Time after time people report to me that as they bring their eating under control, the upsets seem to level out. They are better able to deal with the stress, and they find new solutions to problems that had formerly seemed to overwhelm them. Every part of your body, mind, and spirit functions more effectively when you are sowing to the Spirit.

Question: Couldn't this fasting lead to anorexia?

Answer: This has never been a problem with Scriptural Eating Patterns. The reason is simple: for the first time in their lives, people feel in *control* of their eating!

The word most often used when people describe the difference this teaching has made in their lives is *freedom*. People say, "I feel free for the first time in my life." "My whole life changed as I learned how to sow to the Spirit." A man recently wrote, "My attitude toward food has drastically altered, and my spirits seem to soar as my weight plummets." These are not thoughts and feelings that lead to anorexia.

Personal Inventory or Group Discussion Questions

Chapter One

1. A lot of stress and anxiety in life comes when our ________________ cannot conceive solutions to problems in our lives.

2. In the most difficult and challenging circumstances of life, God asks us to:

- **A.** Lie awake at night and try to figure out an answer.
- **B.** Worry, because worry will ultimately bring a solution.
- **C.** Not allow our hearts to be anxious or troubled.
- **D.** To believe in God and all that He is.

3. Write out John 3:3, John 3:6, and John 6:24.

____

____

____

____

4. Write, in your own words, the difference between your spirit and your flesh. Which one does God work through? ______________________________

____

____

5. Before we are born again, we are subject to ______________________________.

6. *"God is ______________________________, and those who worship Him* [draw close to Him] *must worship in ______________________ and ______________________"* (John 4:24). What do you think that means?

____

____

____

7. When a person is born again, his or her ____________________ comes alive to God.

8. Your freedom and deliverance from compulsive or binge eating comes from:

- **A.** Strict adherence to all the principles in this book.
- **B.** Keeping up with all the latest diets and constantly adjusting what you eat.
- **C.** Your relationship with God.

9. Describe your present relationship with God.

____

____

10. Look up the following verses and describe what they tell about maintaining a healthy, life-giving relationship with God. Give yourself a point value (from 1–10) on each of the areas mentioned: one meaning "almost non-existent in my life" and ten meaning "a regular, consistent part of my relationship with God."

Luke 11:1: *"Now it came to pass, as He was ______________________________ in a certain place."*

Matthew 6:3: *"When you ____________________."*

Matthew 6:6: *"When you ____________________."*

Matthew 6:16: *"When you ____________________."*

Matthew 6:15: *"But if you ______________________ men their trespasses* [willful acts], *neither will your Father __________________ your trespasses."*

Chapter Two

1. What did Jesus say about the flesh in John 6:63? *"The flesh profits ____________________________."*

In your own words, tell what you believe that means. ____

____

____

2. Jesus said that His words are _______________ and ___________________. (See John 6:63.)

3. Dieting is a ____________________ weapon in a ____________________________ battle.

4. List some things that you have tried to control your eating (or other addictive behavior). What has the result been? ______________________________
____
____

5. True or False: Obesity (or gluttony) is mainly a matter of personal vanity.

6. Read the following verses and fill in the spaces.

John 8:32: *"You shall know ____________________, and the truth ________________________________."*
John 8:36: *"Therefore if the Son makes you ______________, you shall be __________________."*

Both of these verses promise us:
- **A.** Control.
- **B.** Struggles.
- **C.** Freedom.
- **D.** A great diet plan.

7. Read Isaiah 61:1–3. List four things that the Spirit of the Lord does by anointing.
- **A.** ____________________
- **B.** ____________________
- **C.** ____________________
- **D.** ____________________

8. What is a "stronghold"? ____________________

____

9. True or False: There is no evidence in Scripture that my binge eating can ever be healed.

10. Has anyone ever told you that your eating problem didn't really matter? ______
Who said it and how did it make you feel?

____

What would you like to say to them?

____

____

Chapter Three

1. What is the *"bread of deceit"* (KJV) spoken of in Proverbs 20:17? ______________________________

____

____

2. What is "soul hunger," and how is it different from just being hungry for food? ________________

____

____

3. Which of these statements are true about anger?

A. Anger is sinful.

B. God will punish those who feel anger toward Him.

C. Anger can hinder healing of food addictions.
D. The best thing to do with anger is to put on a happy face!
E. It doesn't matter what we say when we are angry.
F. Anger is a part of life.
G. Jesus expressed anger.
H. We can be angry at ourselves or others and not even understand why.

4. What is Jesus' invitation when we are *"heavy laden"* (Matthew 11:28) with emotional issues?

"___________________________, all you who labor and are heavy laden, and I will ____________________. Take My ___________ upon you and ____________________ from Me, for I am _____________ and ________________ in heart, and you will find ______________________________" (Matthew 11:28–29).

5. Think about your life and give an example of when you came to Jesus and found rest. What was the result? ____

____

____

6. True or False: God does not care about emotional issues in our lives.

7. Seeds carry ____________________ in them.

8. Define "spiritual intervention." Give an example of a spiritual intervention. ________________

____

____

____

9. How could you make a spiritual intervention in your life with regard to overeating? ____________

____

____

10. True or False: Small fasts are insignificant and won't really help.

11. True or False: Jesus taught us that what we do openly is the most important.

12. True or False: The Bible has a lot to say about gluttony (obsession with food).

13. Complete the following verse:

John 7:17: *"If anyone wants to do His will, he*

____

____."

Read Matthew 7:24–27.
Complete this verse from the reading:

"Whoever hears these sayings of Mine,

____,

I will liken him to a __________ *man"* (Matthew 7:24).

Chapter Four

1. What was God's original plan for eating (Genesis 2:16)?

"Of every tree of the garden, you may ______________ ______________."

2. How does your relationship with food compare with this original freedom? ____________________

____

____

3. What are some of the ideas that you have formed about food that you are now reevaluating because of what you are learning? ______________

____

____

4. Look up Exodus 16:12 and 1 Kings 14:4–6. What do these two examples have in common?

____

____

____

5. True or False: God was establishing an inflexible law in these verses that we must always try to follow.

6. True or False: Eating two meals a day is the secret of being freed from food addictions.

7. What is a key question to ask yourself before you eat anything? ______________________________

____

8. What natural responses did God put in man to balance out his eating? _________________ and

___________.

9. True or False: Hunger is a painful response that lasts for hours and hours.

10. True or False: Digesting food is a quick and easy process for the body, and it is a good idea to eat a big meal when you want to function at peak performance.

11. What, if anything, can a person do to help these natural controls take over again? ________________

____

____

12. In the parable of the sower found in Mark 4, what three things choke out the word?

A. _____________________

B. _____________________

C. _____________________

13. In that same parable, what do we discover is necessary to have in ourselves in order for the seed to grow?

___________________ provide stability, nourishment, and moisture to a plant.

14. What do you think the illustration of the root represented? ______________________________

____

____

15. More than anything else, the healing process comes about by

A. A strict adherence to an eating plan, such as two meals a day.
B. Fasting one meal.
C. Developing a daily relationship that brings the power of God into my eating.

Chapter Five

1. True or False: God has a purpose and a good plan for *my* life.

2. God sometimes gives gifts of ______________ in regard to situations in our lives.

3. True or False: The best way to bring healing into my life is to "go with the flow" and just let my day happen.

4. Fill in this verse: "_________________ *the path of your feet and let all your ways* ____________________________" (Proverbs 4:26).

5. Define the two key words in this verse. Use a dictionary.

A. ponder ____________________________
B. establish ___________________________

6. How do these words apply to eating? _______

____

____

7. What is the benefit of thinking about and writing down certain activities as substitutes for eating? ___________________________________

____

____

8. Our brains tend to develop new habits in cycles of:

30 days   7 days   21 days   2 months

9. True or False: If I binge eat again, it means that I can't be healed.

10. What does the Bible call Satan?
"The ____________________ of our brethren" (Revelation 12:10).

11. What type of thoughts does Satan try to plant in our minds? ______________________________

____

____

12. List several thoughts that you believe he has repeatedly tried to plant in your mind.

____

____

____

____

13. When I speak something out loud, I benefit because I can ______________ it as well as think it or read it.

14. True or False: We can develop habits in regard to eating that we are not even conscious of.

Chapter Six

1. Write out Proverbs 13:2 and Proverbs 18:20:

____

____

____

____

____

What do both of these verses talk about? The ________________ of his _____________.

2. Read Philippians 4:7–8 and write down the things that are healthy to think about. __________

____

____

____

3. Read Philippians 4:9: *"The things which you __________________ and ___________________ and __________________ and _________________ in me, these ______________, and the God of _______________ will be _______________________."*

4. True or False: It doesn't matter what I think about.

5. One way to change what I think is to change what I ____________________________________.

6. Write down at least three thoughts that you can read or speak to bring you hope. These can be Scriptures, paraphrases of Scriptures, or just words that are based on truth.

A. ____________________________________

____

B. ____________________________________

____

C. ____________________________________

____

7. True or False: The fruit of my mouth is nourishment to my soul.

Chapter Seven

1. Read Genesis 2:16. *"Of every tree of the garden, you may ______________________________________."*

2. True or False: Jesus said that we should be very, very cautious about what we eat.

3. What instructions did Jesus give the seventy disciples that He sent out? (See Luke 10:7–8.)

____

____

4. According to Matthew 15:11, what defiles a man? __________________________________

____

5. What advice did Paul give with regard to different ideas about what people should or should not eat? (See Colossians 2:20.) ____________________

____

6. True or False: The Bible often condemns eating sweets.

7. *"________________________ does not commend us to God"* (1 Corinthians 8:8).

8. What is "junk food"? ____________________

____

9. What are some words that clue us in to "junk foods"?

________________flavor
________________ coloring
less than ______% actual fruit juice

10. Why is it a bad idea to eat many of these "foods"?

They deprive our ____________________ of ____.

11. Which best describes what our attitude should be about these foods?

A. It is a sin to eat such foods.
B. It is unwise to each such non-foods.

12. List five foods that you tend to feel guilty about eating.

A. ____
B. ____
C. ____
D. ____
E. ____

13. What kind of influence does that feeling of guilt over these foods cause?

A. I feel as if I have blown it when I eat these foods, so I overeat other things, as well.
B. I feel as if I have done wrong when I eat these foods.
C. I tend to overeat them when I do allow myself to have them.
D. I usually don't eat them, but I often can't stop thinking about them when I don't eat them.

Chapter Eight

1. Read 1 Timothy 4:4–5. What happens to our food when we pray over it? *"It is* ________________ *by the word of God and prayer"* (v. 5).

2. What does the word *"sanctified"* mean? ______

____

____

3. Jesus gave us a strong example by ___________ over His food.

4. When are you least likely to pray over your food?

- **A.** When I am sitting down to eat with my family
- **B.** When I am alone
- **C.** In a restaurant with friends
- **D.** At holiday dinners
- **E.** While binge eating

5. When should we pray over our food? _______

____

____

6. What can happen when you pray over something you are going to eat? __________________

____

____

Discussion Questions

Chapters 9 & 10

1. Our bodies ______________ through the years. A person uses ____________ calories as he grows older.

2. True or false: A person can gain weight in middle age without changing what he is eating.

3. Statistically speaking, people who do vigorous exercise for __________ minutes a day, __________ times a week are ___________ percent less likely to develop every disease.

4. Name some of the benefits of incorporating regular exercise into your life choices:

____

____

5. Jesus said, *"He who is ____________________ in what is least is __________________ also in much"* (Luke 16:10).

6. What does that verse tell us about the danger of little compromises? ______________________

____

____

7. What does that verse tell us about the value of small victories? ________________________

____

____

8. Can you give an example in your own life of a big battle that was won with small victories?

___

___

9. Name seven (or more) areas of vulnerability that a person needs to keep track of:
(roadblocks to healing)

1.
2.
3.
4.
5.
6.
7.
Other:

Answers to Discussion Questions

Chapter 1

1. minds
2. C, D
3. John 3:3; John 3:6; John 6:24
4. Flesh is temporal; spirit is eternal. Flesh is weak; spirit is strong. God is Spirit and works through our spirits.
5. bondage
6. a spirit; spirit; truth; (in your own words)
7. spirit
8. C
9. (in your own words)
10. praying, do a charitable deed, pray, fast, do not forgive, forgive; (in your own words)

Chapter 2

1. nothing; (your own words expressing frustration of fighting flesh with flesh, for example, dieting doesn't produce lasting change.)
2. spirit; life
3. carnal, fleshly; spiritual
4. (in your own words)
5. False
6. the truth, shall set you free; free, free indeed; C

7. A. preaches good tidings (give real hope)
   B. binds up the brokenhearted
   C. proclaims liberty to the captives
   D. opens prison to them that are bound
8. An unbreakable habit; something that has a "strong hold" on an area of your life.
9. False
10. (in your own words)

Chapter 3

1. Food eaten for emotional reasons or reasons other than hunger.
2. Soul hunger originates from our emotions or our souls. It cannot be satisfied by food, and so, eating food, instead of dealing with the emotional need, results in an insatiable intake of food that does not satisfy.
3. C, F, G, H
4. Come to Me, give you rest, yoke, learn, gentle, lowly, rest for your souls.
5. (in your own words)
6. False
7. life
8. A spiritual intervention is when a person deliberately changes his physical circumstances for a spiritual purpose; (in your own words).
9. Change my location; change my activity (or lack of activity), change my solitude to being with people—and "do" it as a seed of obedience sown in secret before God.
10. False
11. False

12. True
13. will know of the doctrine, whether it is of God; and does them, wise

Chapter 4

1. freely eat
2. (in your own words)
3. (in your own words); example: "Some foods are bad and wrong to eat. I feel guilty when I eat them."
4. God is supernaturally feeding. He feeds twice a day (morning and evening).
5. False
6. False
7. Am I really hungry?
8. Hunger and fullness
9. False
10. False
11. Allow your body to become hungry before you eat. Be aware of your body's full response. Get to know "hunger"; how it works, how long it lasts, etc. Get to know "full"; how quickly does it come? What happens when you continue eating?
12. A. cares of this world
    B. deceitfulness of riches
    C. lust for other things
13. Roots
14. The necessity of maintaining our spiritual relationship with God through prayer, fasting, giving, and reading His Word.
15. C

Chapter 5

1. True
2. wisdom or knowledge
3. False
4. Ponder, be established
5. Answer from dictionary.
6. Give thought and attention to what you are doing and eating. Have a plan. "Ponder."
7. It helps to break the habit of overeating.
8. 21 days
9. False
10. accuser
11. Self-hatred, defeat, hopelessness, judgment
12. (in your own words)
13. hear
14. True

Chapter 6

1. Proverbs 13:2; Proverbs 18:20; "fruit," mouth
2. (Philippians 4:7–8 in your own words)
3. learned, received, heard, saw, do, peace, with you
4. False
5. say
6. (in your own words)
7. True

Chapter 7

1. freely eat
2. False
3. Eat and drink whatever is served to you.

4. That which comes out of the mouth (from the heart).
5. Don't be "subject to regulations"; don't get off track by making too big a deal out of what you eat. Maintain the freedom you have in Christ.
6. False
7. Food
8. "Pretend" food that has undergone so much processing that it is no longer "food" that nourishes our bodies and satisfies our hunger.
9. artificial, artificial, 10%
10. bodies, real nutrition that they need to function in a healthy way.
11. B
12. (in your own words)
13. All of the answers are correct. A, B, C, D

Chapter 8

1. sanctified
2. Made holy; freed from sin.
3. praying (blessing it, giving thanks to God for it)
4. (in your own words)
5. Whenever we eat, especially when we are alone.
6. As you pray, you can receive help from God that is so powerful that you will not eat the food that you were going to eat for the wrong reasons.

Chapters 9 & 10

1. change; fewer
2. True
3. 20; 3; 50

4. A. Muscle uses 30% more calories than fat.
   B. Helps maintain flexibility.
   C. Helps maintain muscle tone
   D. Reduces the risk of all diseases by 50%
   E. Promotes emotional stability
   F. Decreases stress
5. Faithful, faithful
6. They can lead to bigger problems.
7. Small victories are the road to BIG, lifelong victories.
8. (in your own words)
9. 1. Trying to take on the whole problem instead of living one day at a time, one small victory at a time.
   2. Getting back into the "diet syndrome" by restricting certain foods and feeling guilty about eating them.
   3. Knowingly sowing to the flesh; deliberately choosing a situation that leads to overeating.
   4. Leaving the house (soul, spirit) empty. Not maintaining a vital relationship with God.
   5. Sowing from abundance rather than from your want. This happens when our relationship with God becomes habit rather than hunger for Him.
   6. Sowing in a hit-or-miss manner.
   7. Not being faithful with the seed you have decided to sow. Not keeping a secret vow to God—whatever it is. God hears our vows. God expects us to keep them. It is much better to make a small commitment and keep it than to make a big one and not keep it.

Scriptures

Proverbs

The drunkard and the glutton will come to poverty. (23:21)

Bread gained by deceit is sweet to a man, but afterward his mouth will be filled with gravel. (20:17)

Do not desire...delicacies, for they are deceptive food. (23:3)

Ponder [think about] *the path of your feet, and let all your ways be established.* (4:26)

A satisfied soul loathes the honeycomb, but to a hungry soul every bitter thing is sweet. (27:7)

My son, let them [God's words] *not depart from your eyes; keep sound wisdom and discretion* [the ability to choose]*; so they will be life to your soul and grace to your neck.* (3:21–22)

The fear of the LORD is the beginning of wisdom, and the knowledge of the Holy One is understanding. (9:10)

New Testament

The kingdom of God is not eating and drinking, but righteousness and peace and joy in the Holy Spirit. (Romans 14:17)

The thief does not come except to steal, and to kill, and to destroy. I have come that they may have life, and that they may have it more abundantly.
(John 10:10)

The kingdom of heaven is like a mustard seed, which a man took and sowed in his field. (Matthew 13:31)

Some fell on stony ground, where it did not have much earth; and immediately it sprang up because it had no depth of earth. But when the sun was up it was scorched, and because it had no root it withered away....These likewise are the ones sown on stony ground who, when they hear the word, immediately receive it with gladness; and they have no root in themselves, and so endure only for a time.
(Mark 4:5–6, 16–17)

The cares of this world, the deceitfulness of riches, and the desires for other things...choke the word, and it becomes unfruitful. (Mark 4:19)

But the fruit of the Spirit is love, joy, peace, longsuffering, kindness, goodness, faithfulness, gentleness, self-control. Against such there is no law.
(Galations 5:22–23)

Do not be decieved, God is not mocked; for whatever a man sows, that he will also reap. (Galatians 6:7)

Come to Me, all you who labor and are heavy laden, and I will give you rest. Take My yoke upon you and learn from Me, for I am gentle and lowly in heart, and you will find rest for your souls. For My yoke is easy and My burden is light. (Matthew 11:28–30)

About the Author

Diane Hampton has traveled all over the country and abroad, teaching the Bible and ministering to people who are hurting. She is the first female vice president of Teen Challenge in St. Louis, a drug and alcohol rehabilitation program. She currently travels with Service International, a Christian humanitarian organization that helps to build shelters, aid in flood relief, and provide help in times of crisis in such places as Kosovo and Zimbabwe, as well as the States. Every Sunday for the last five years, Diane has taught the Scriptures at the West County Assembly of God in St. Louis. She has recently started a custom greeting card line, incorporating her love for both photography and God's creation. Diane and her husband, Don, have been married for thirty-seven years and have two daughters.

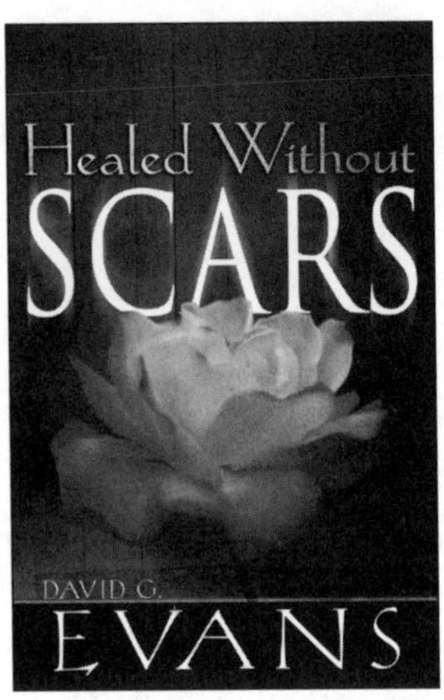

Healed Without Scars
David G. Evans

Have you been hurt by past disappointment, fear, rejection, abandonment, or failure? If so, you've probably learned that time doesn't necessarily heal all wounds. When pain from the past lingers in our lives and causes emotional scars, you need to understand that God is always ready to help you! Discover the path to personal wholeness, and find peace in the midst of life's storms. Renew your hopes and dreams, and experience a life of freedom and joy. For years, author David Evans has helped people from all walks of life learn how to live in victory. Let him guide you to a joyful life of wholeness in Christ as you learn that you can be *Healed Without Scars*!

ISBN: 978-0-88368-542-2 • Trade • 272 pages

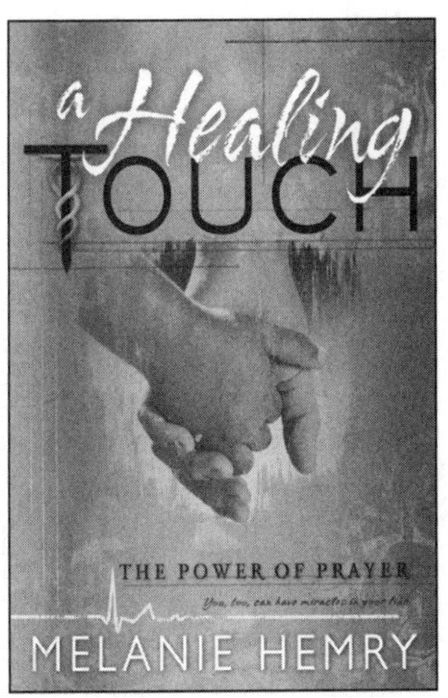

A Healing Touch: The Power of Prayer

Melanie Hemry

We all want prayers that move the hand of God. We want to be used and blessed and effective for the kingdom of God. But when someone says "intercessor," we balk, we run, we thank God that it's not our gift or our calling....But it is.

Melanie Hemry will challenge everything you ever believed about prayer. She will introduce you to a new kind of prayer—the soul-stirring, world-shaking, life-giving *prayer* that this world so desperately needs. As a former ICU nurse and prayer warrior, Melanie is qualified to give you the heart transplant you need. You will not walk away from this book unchanged.

ISBN: 978-0-88368-780-2 • Trade • 192 pages

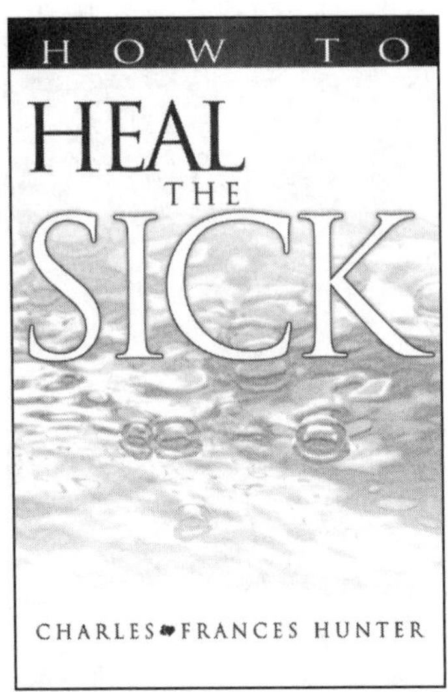

How to Heal the Sick

Charles and Frances Hunter

A loved one is sick...your friend was just in an accident...a family member is facing an emotional crisis. Have you ever desperately longed to reach out your hand and bring healing to these needs? At times our hearts ache with the desire to help, but either we don't know how or we are afraid and stop short. The truth is that, as a Christian, the Holy Spirit within you is ready to heal the sick! Charles and Frances Hunter present solid, biblically based methods of healing that can bring not only physical health, but also spiritual wholeness and the abundant life to you, your family, and everyone around you.

ISBN: 978-0-88368-600-3 • Trade • 224 pages

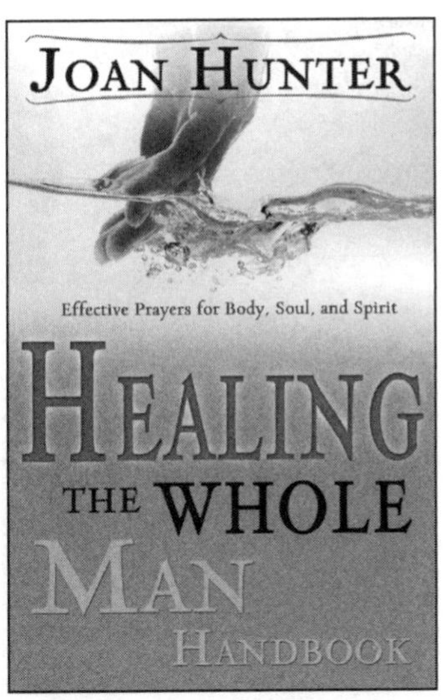

Healing the Whole Man Handbook: Effective Prayers for Body, Soul, and Spirit

Joan Hunter

You can walk in divine health and healing. The secrets to God's words for healing and recovery are in this comprehensive, easy-to-follow guidebook containing powerful healing prayers that cover everything from abuse to yeast infections and everything in between.

Truly anointed with the gifts of healing, Joan Hunter has over thirty years of experience praying for the sick and brokenhearted and seeing them healed and set free. By following these step-by-step instructions and claiming God's promises, you can be healed, set free, and made totally whole—body, soul, and spirit!

ISBN: 978-0-88368-815-8 • Trade • 240 pages

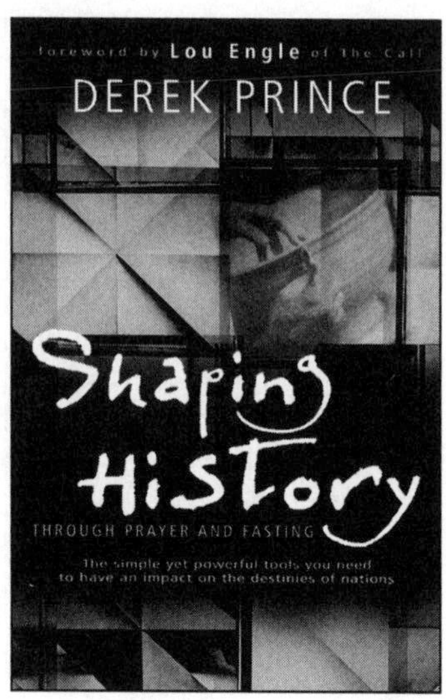

Shaping History through Prayer and Fasting
Derek Prince

The times we are living in are scary, to say the least, yet what we are facing isn't new. History is replete with violent episodes of unimaginable carnage and terror. And what did people do about them? The only thing they could do—they prayed! Best-selling author Derek Prince reveals how your prayers can make a real difference right now and into the future. Discover how to touch the heart of God through effective fasting and prayer—prayer that will change the world!

ISBN: 978-0-88368-773-4 • Trade • 192 pages

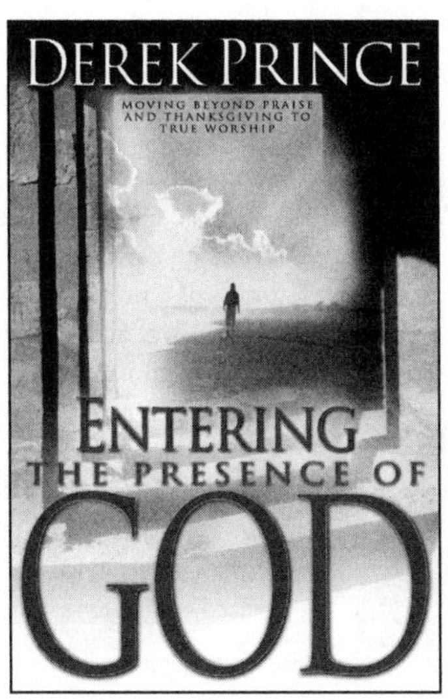

Entering the Presence of God
Derek Prince

"The harder I try to be good, the worse off I am!" If that sounds like you, there's good news. Internationally acclaimed Bible teacher Derek Prince shows the way to victorious intimacy with God as he explains how you can enter into His very presence to receive the spiritual, physical, and emotional blessings of true worship. Learn the secrets of entering into the Lord's rest, fellowshipping with the Father, receiving revelation from God's Spirit, and conducting spiritual warfare. Discover how to be freed from the bondage of guilt and sin and obtain an inner peace and joy that nothing else can duplicate. Don't miss out on the thrill of worship...God's way!

ISBN: 978-0-88368-719-2 • Trade • 176 pages

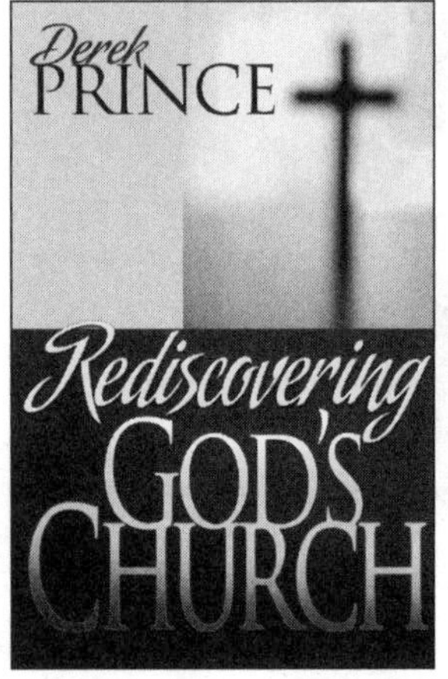

Rediscovering God's Church

Derek Prince

What is God's original blueprint for the church? How can you discover your place in His plan? Derek Prince answers these questions and many others as he describes God's true intention for the body of Christ. The church is God's family: a place of love, acceptance, joy, and learning; a refuge from the stresses of the world, an oasis where you are strengthened in your walk with the Lord. Any church can become increasingly alive if we allow the Spirit to infuse us with a new sense of His purpose. Become an active participant in your local community of believers by *Rediscovering God's Church*!

ISBN: 978-0-88368-812-0 • Hardcover • 432 pages

Appointment in Jerusalem
30th Anniversary Edition

Derek and Lydia Prince

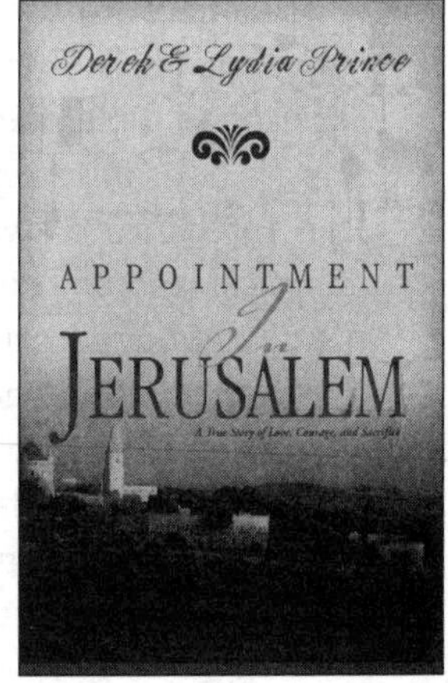

Here is the riveting true story of a young schoolteacher and her courageous quest to know God's will for her life. In Lydia Prince's search for God and her life's purpose, she is led to Jerusalem where she learns the power of prayer and experiences many miracles of provision and protection. Lydia survives many dangers, including gunfire, siege, and barricades. She enters into her true appointment from God and, in the process, rescues scores of abandoned sick and orphaned children from disease and death. Discover how God can remarkably use those who trust Him!

ISBN: 978-0-88368-794-9 • Hardcover • 304 pages

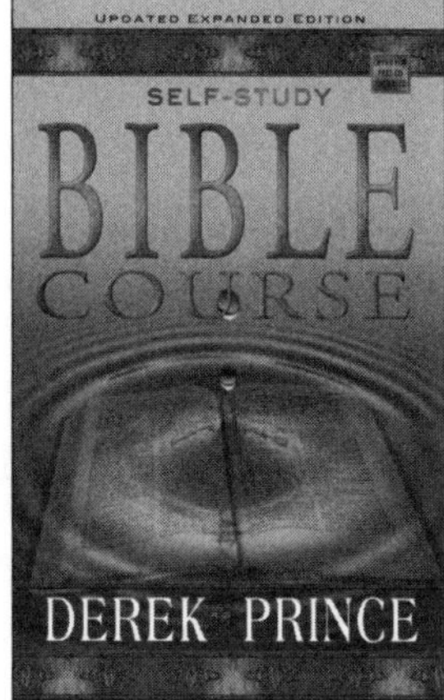

Self-Study Bible Course, Expanded Edition

Derek Prince

If you have questions about God and the Bible, here is the help you need. In this Bible study course, you will find answers to questions such as, "How can I have victory over sin?" and "How can I receive answers to my prayers?" If you have never read the Bible before, you will find this systematic study guide easy to use and helpful. Or, if you have been a believer for many years, you will find a new ease in conversing with God, fellowshipping with Christians, and witnessing and winning souls. This expanded edition provides an in-depth exploration of topics such as healing and guidance.

ISBN: 978-0-88368-750-5 • Workbook • 216 pages

Lucifer Exposed

Derek Prince

The fall of Lucifer set up the epic "battle of the ages." And you are positioned right in the midst of this historic struggle. Satan, the fallen archangel, desires nothing more than to win the loyalty, hearts, and minds of the entire human race—and he won't quit in his attempt to win you over! In *Lucifer Exposed*, Derek Prince uncovers Satan's greatest weapon in enslaving the average human into bondage. Satan attempts to seduce Christians from rising to their full potential and to distract every human being from following God. Use the mighty spiritual warfare weapons revealed in this compelling book, and victory can be yours!

ISBN: 978-0-88368-836-6 • Trade • 224 pages

www.whitakerhouse.com